HOW TO PREVENT FOOD POISONING

HOW TO PREVENT FOOD POISONING

A Practical Guide to Safe Cooking, Eating, and Food Handling

Elizabeth Scott, Ph.D.
Paul Sockett, Ph.D.

John Wiley & Sons, Inc.

New York • Chichester • Weinheim • Brisbane • Singapore • Toronto

Published by John Wiley & Sons, Inc.
Published simultaneously in Canada

This publication is designed to provide accurate and authoritative information in regard to the subject matter covered. It is sold with the understanding that the publisher is not engaged in rendering professional services. If professional advice or other expert assistance is required, the services of a competent professional person should be sought.

Library of Congress Cataloging-in-Publication Data:
Scott, Elizabeth
     How to prevent food poisoning : a practical guide to safe cooking, eating, and food handling / Elizabeth Scott, Paul Sockett.
         p.   cm.
     Includes index.
     ISBN: 978-1-62045-691-0
     1. Food handling.   2. Food contamination.   3. Food poisoning--Prevention.   I. Sockett, Paul   II. Title.
TX537.S38   1998
363.19'26--dc21   97-49025
                                                                              CIP

For our families

Andrew, Raoul, Loren, and Joshua
—E. S.

Rosemarie, Fiona, Lisa, and Philip
—P. S.

CONTENTS

Acknowledgments   xiii

Introduction   1

PART ONE
WHAT IS FOOD POISONING?   5

1 THE RISE OF FOOD POISONING   7

The Iceberg Effect   8

2 WHAT CAUSES FOOD POISONING?   11

Chemicals   12
Solid Objects   13
Naturally Occurring Poisons   14
Germs and Parasitic Worms   15
Allergies and Food Intolerance   20
Growth and Multiplication of Bacteria   20

3 EGGS, HAMBURGERS, BERRIES, WATER, AND MAD COW DISEASE   26

Salmonella   26
Hamburger Disease: *E. Coli*   27

Diarrhea and Berries   28
Watery Problems   28
Mad Cow Disease   29
Antibiotic Resistance and Food
    Poisoning Germs   31

PART TWO
FOOD POISONING AND YOU   35

4   SYMPTOMS AND COMPLICATIONS OF
     FOOD POISONING   37

     Common Symptoms and Their Severity   37
     Complications of Food Poisoning   39
     Who Gets Food Poisoning?   42

5   WHAT TO DO IF YOU GET FOOD POISONING   48

PART THREE
HOW TO PREVENT FOOD POISONING
WHEN SHOPPING   51

6   CHOOSING WHERE TO SHOP FOR FOOD   53

     Visual Clues for a Safe Food Store   53
     How to Become a Revolting Consumer   54

Contents

7 SHOPPING FOR FOOD 57

Selecting Fresh Meat 57
Selecting Fresh Seafood 60
Shopping for Fresh Produce 61
Shopping from Delis, Salad Bars, and Bakeries 62
Shopping for Refrigerated and Frozen Foods 65
Shopping for Canned, Dried, and Bottled Foods 68

8 THE CHECK-OUT AND GETTING THE FOOD HOME SAFELY 71

PART FOUR
HOW TO PREVENT FOOD POISONING IN YOUR KITCHEN 73

9 STORING FOOD AT HOME 75

Refrigerated and Frozen Foods 75
Canned, Bottled, and Dried Foods 79
Fruits and Vegetables 79
Breads and Pastries 80
Deciding When to Reject Food 80

10 PREPARING AND COOKING FOOD SAFELY 82

Raw Foods of Animal Origin 82
Preventing Cross-Contamination 83
Eggs 84
Cooking Food to Make It Safe 84

Safety Tips for Cooking   86
Tasting the Safe Way   88
Making Recipes Safe   88
Cooking on the Grill   89
Microwave Cooking   90

11   SERVING FOOD SAFELY AND DEALING
     WITH LEFTOVERS   93

Serving a Safe Buffet   94
Dealing with Leftovers   95

12   COOKING FOR HOLIDAYS AND PARTIES   98

The Big Holiday Meal   99
Parties at Home   100

13   HOME FOOD PRESERVATION   103

Botulism   104
Preservation Techniques   105

14   KITCHEN DESIGN AND SANITATION   111

Planning a Kitchen and Choosing Equipment   111
Hygienic Handwashing   114
Cleaning and Sanitizing in the Kitchen   115

PART FIVE
SAFE COOKING FOR SPECIAL NEEDS 119

15 COOKING FOR HIGHER-RISK INDIVIDUALS 121

What Foods Should Higher-Risk Individuals
    Avoid? 121
How to Cook for a Higher-Risk Individual 122
Dietary Factors that Can Increase the Risk of
    Foodborne Illness 123

16 COOKING FOR SENIORS AND SINGLES 126

PART SIX
SAFE EATING AWAY FROM HOME 131

17 HOW TO AVOID FOOD POISONING À LA CARTE 133

Pointers to Safe Food Restaurants and Take-Outs 133
Traveling Abroad 137
Eating Safely at Campsites, Picnics, and Potlucks 138
Camping 138
Picnics 139
Preparing and Cooking for Potlucks and Nonprofit
    Events 141

PART SEVEN

THE SCIENCE OF FOOD POISONING   143

18   HOW FOOD POISONING GERMS MAKE YOU ILL   145

The Body's Defenses Against Food Poisoning   145
The Human Digestive Passage   146
The Germ   148
Type 1: Poison (Toxin) Produced in the Food   150
Type 2: Poison (Toxin) Released in the Intestines   152
Type 3: Infection in the Intestines   153
Type 4: Infection in the Blood and Body Organs   154
The Food   155

PART EIGHT

SELF-ASSESSMENT   157

19   FOOD SAFETY QUIZ   159

Test Your Knowledge of How to Prevent Food
   Poisoning   159

APPENDIX   165
The Rogues' Gallery: An A-Z Guide to Food Poisoning
   Germs   165
Bacteria   165
Viruses   181
Parasites   184
Seafood Toxins   188

Glossary   191

Bibliography   195

Index   197

ACKNOWLEDGMENTS

We wish to thank the many friends and colleagues on both sides of the Atlantic who have supported and encouraged us in the writing of this book. Many people have answered our questions with a generosity of time and enthusiasm. You are anonymous, but you know who you are and we thank you.

We thank our literary agent, Bill Adler, himself a survivor of a life-threatening encounter with *Salmonella* food poisoning, for making contact with us in the first place, and for his help and encouragement in preparing the proposal for this book. We thank Fiona Sockett for her ideas for illustrations and for preparing the drawing that appears in the book. We also thank Dr. Jeff Farber of Health Canada and Laurie M. Malcom and Tracy Geran, Sanitary Inspectors in Newton, Massachusetts, for their technical advice.

Final thanks go to our editor, Tom Miller, who not only took on the task of bringing together our two different styles but also offered many valuable ideas and patiently showed us how to craft our first book, and to his assistant, Elaine O'Neal.

INTRODUCTION

When Sheila rushed her young baby into the emergency room suffering from severe vomiting, dehydration, and fits, her only concern was for the recovery of her child. Later, after three days of worry, she began to wonder how the baby had become ill and why it was the only member of the family to do so.

The illness suffered by Sheila's baby was not an isolated incident. Scientists believe that each year millions of people in industrialized countries such as the United States, the United Kingdom, Australia, and Japan succumb to food poisoning. The toll is probably even higher in developing countries where hygiene and sanitation are poorer than that found in industrialized nations. Big outbreaks of food poisoning make headlines like KILLER BUG IN YOUR FOOD and HUNDREDS ILL IN FOOD SCARE, but as many as half of all cases are part of a quiet epidemic that repeats itself in many of our homes every year. Much of this illness could be prevented.

Food poisoning is costly in many ways. The physical and emotional costs are painful. Most people suffer a few days of discomfort, inconvenience, and lost work or school. A smaller but significant number develop more severe forms of illness and are admitted to a hospital. Still others experience long-term disability or even die. In addition, the financial costs of illness cannot be ignored: for just one victim, medical costs, loss of work, home help costs, and so forth could run into the thousands of dollars.

While it is in the best interests of food manufacturers to make every effort to ensure that our food is safe to eat, through the application of good practices in production, transport, and retailing, it is currently not possible to guarantee this 100 percent. National and local governments also try to protect our food supplies through food production and food hygiene legislation and codes of safe practice, through inspection and enforcement, monitoring, education, and research, but may be frustrated by the

1

limitation of resources available to them. It seems that almost every year a new "bug" appears or a new risk is identified. In the past few years alone there has been a steady stream of media reports about big outbreaks of *Salmonella* food poisoning or "new" food poisoning germs such as *E. coli,* which caused the "hamburger disease," and BSE, the cause of "mad cow disease."

With all the media reports of *Salmonella* food poisoning and of children dying from hamburger disease, you'd think that everyone would be making an effort to prevent these outbreaks and tragedies. Yet our combined experience, which covers over thirty-five years of research into food poisoning and food hygiene, shows that people preparing food go on making the same mistakes— allowing raw food to contaminate kitchen surfaces and cooked food, storing ready-to-eat food too long at room temperature, or simply failing to wash their hands after a visit to the toilet. Next time you visit a public toilet, note how many people leave without washing their hands—one of those people could be going to work in the restaurant where you're about to lunch.

From conversations we've had with consumer groups and on televised talk shows, we know that people are concerned about food safety but that they either do not understand the causes of food poisoning or don't know how to put their knowledge into practice, especially in the home situation. It is for this reason that we wrote this book. We felt it was important both to give an easy-to-read account of how food poisoning happens and to provide a step-by-step guide to safe shopping, preparation, cooking, and storage of food in everyday home situations.

We know that there are a host of reasons why people don't follow basic food hygiene rules. Some may simply lack knowledge or be unwilling to believe that the things they've done for the last thirty years are risky, or they're "too busy to take the time." For others, it may be a matter of beliefs or attitude or simply space considerations ("My kitchen is just too small to stick to the rules"). In reality, these are excuses not reasons. This book gives practical guidelines that are an easy addition to everyone's food-handling skills. These guidelines do not require a lot of extra time or fuss, they do not require a special kitchen, and it is never too late to learn new skills.

The last line of defense against most food poisoning is the person who buys, prepares, and cooks the food. This book is therefore specifically aimed at anyone who prepares food in the home, whether for themselves or for their family and friends. We have divided the book into sections that describe food poisoning and how specific germs make people sick. We talk about some of the current concerns in food safety, and most important, we take you through all the aspects of safe purchase, transport, preparation, and storage of food. Whenever necessary, we address specific concerns of people at higher risk of developing severe illness, including the very young, the elderly, those with serious existing illnesses such as cancer and leukemia, and those with damaged immune systems caused by infections such as AIDS or by treatment with chemotherapy.

Read each section independently, or read the entire book for a more complete and detailed understanding of food poisoning and how to prevent it. Whatever your approach, we would encourage you to check out the sections on safe food handling in Parts Three and Four. When you've done that, test yourself by working through the quiz in Chapter 19 and see how much you've learned. Above all, we urge you to put your knowledge into practice in your own kitchen. We cannot guarantee that you'll never get food poisoning, but you certainly could reduce the risk and prevent unnecessary illness to yourself and your family in the future.

PART ONE

WHAT IS FOOD POISONING?

1

THE RISE OF FOOD POISONING

Headlines warning of a "killer bug" in hamburgers, chicken, cheese, salad, or fruit seem to be common fare these days. No headlines, however, could have prepared Maureen and Jim for the personal anguish of watching their previously healthy daughter struggling to survive kidney failure as her little body was ravaged by the so-called "hamburger disease"—the tragic outcome of eating an undercooked hamburger served at a party five days earlier. After a stormy three weeks, Maureen and Jim are left counting the cost of an illness that should never have occurred. Their family life has been turned upside-down and from now on will revolve around their daughter's need for regular kidney dialysis. Coupled with this is the desperate hope of a kidney transplant and the worry about its success. Their main concern at the moment is for their daughter's recovery, but they will soon need to focus on the financial costs of treatment and convalescence and on the disruption to their lives and careers.

Sadly, such stories appear all too frequently in newspapers and magazines and on talk shows, reflecting public concern over what should be a preventable disease. They also illustrate the potential seriousness of food poisoning. Although most victims experience only a few days of inconvenience and discomfort, others progress to life-threatening complications and long-term disability—and some die.

In addition to the miserable physical symptoms, food poisoning can be costly in terms of medical bills, missed work opportunities, canceled arrangements, and spoiled holidays. Personal costs can also include such things as replacing soiled clothing and bedding, buying extra disinfectant and cleaning materials, and employing home help as needed. Studies show that these costs are borne not only by the person who was ill but often by other family members and even by friends.

THE ICEBERG EFFECT

Food poisoning is found worldwide and is an important cause of human illness just about everywhere. In nonindustrialized countries, food poisoning and other diarrhea diseases are a major cause of illness and death, particularly in young children. Unfortunately, adequate systems for reporting and recording these cases do not exist in most of those countries.

Reports from many industrialized countries suggest that food poisoning cases are either on the increase or are simply being reported in high numbers. In the United States, for example, as many as twenty thousand cases are officially recorded each year. In the United Kingdom, reported cases of food poisoning increased by 400 percent between 1985, when about twenty thousand cases were recorded, and 1996, when numbers had risen to about eighty thousand. These figures were probably the result of (1) increased awareness, which led to more cases being reported, and (2) a real growth in the number of cases.

But the official figures for food poisoning are only the tip of a very large iceberg. Public health scientists in the United States estimate that each year up to 30 million people get food poisoning and as many as nine thousand deaths are linked to it—quite a difference from the official statistics of twenty thousand recorded cases. Why? Quite simply, most cases are not reported to a public health authority. Most people do not seek medical help for what appears to be a mild stomach upset—an illness that may have been caused by something they ate.

Staggering Statistics

Each day in the United States, an estimated sixteen thousand people become ill with food poisoning, and twenty-five people die, mostly children or the elderly, from illnesses they contract from food poisoning.

Headlines such as the following grab attention when major outbreaks of food poisoning affect large numbers of people or cause serious illness or death.

E. coli Alert
Can This Meat Kill You?
Millions May Be Eating Themselves Sick
The Strawberry Sickness
Fruit Juices Linked to E. coli Outbreak
School Food Scare

Most recently, a spate of "hamburger disease" outbreaks have hit the headlines in North America, the United Kingdom, Australia, and Japan. Outbreaks of E. coli, such as those linked to Jack In The Box fast-food restaurants in the United States in 1996, and those in Scotland in 1997, have shaken public confidence in the safety of the food supply. The public has also been warned about Salmonella on meat, fruit, eggs, and bean sprouts, and about a new threat, Cyclospora, the single-celled parasite that has been found on raspberries. One of the biggest food poisoning outbreaks documented in the United States was in Minnesota in 1985, when an estimated two hundred thousand people were affected by Sal-

monella gastroenteritis after drinking contaminated milk from a single dairy.

In the United Kingdom, the most ominous threat of recent years is the link between bovine spongiform encephalopathy (BSE) in cattle and a deadly new form of the brain-destroying Creutzfeldt-Jakob disease (CJD). At the present time, it is difficult for public health officials to predict how many people will be affected, but the possibility that many people have been exposed to contaminated meat cannot be ignored.

Besides these big outbreaks, which are usually linked to a widely distributed food product, the information available to scientists suggests that as many as half of all cases of food poisoning in the United States result from eating contaminated food prepared in the home. But whether the illness occurs after eating in the home or after eating out, it usually results from mistakes made during the preparation or storage of the food, and in many instances, *it could have been prevented.*

This book is about preventing food poisoning in the home by identifying how and why mistakes occur and following simple guidelines to help avoid illness.

2

WHAT CAUSES
FOOD POISONING?

The term "food poisoning" is used to describe any illness that results from ingesting contaminated food or drink. Unfortunately, most people will experience some sort of food poisoning several times during their lifetime. Most will recover after a few days, but for some people, the illness may last for weeks or months. Symptoms can be severe and may even cause death. (Common symptoms and complications of food poisoning are described in detail in Chapter 4.)

The good news is that most food poisoning is preventable, and the key to prevention is understanding how food becomes a potential source of danger. Here are the main reasons that food and drink can sometimes be unsafe:

- Chemical contamination
- Contamination with solid objects
- The presence of naturally occurring poisons
- Contamination by germs and parasitic worms
- Allergic reactions

CHEMICALS

> ***Golden Rule:*** Empty chemical containers should never be used to store food, drink, or medicines.

Unwanted chemicals may get into food or drink at any stage during production, processing, and preparation. Accidents and carelessness are the usual culprits, but deliberate acts of sabotage also occur.

Common Causes of Chemical Contamination

  • *Pesticides and herbicides are inappropriately or carelessly used during growth of the food.*
  • *Spillage of disinfectant or cleaning substances occurs during preparation and processing of food or drink.*
  • *Substances within food-container materials dissolve into food or drink during storage.*
  • *Wrongly labeled substances are mistakenly added to food and drink during processing and preparation.*

Chemical contaminants may alter the taste or smell of food or drink to the point where it is unpalatable to humans. When this happens, the affected items are usually thrown out before they can do any harm. For example, if a strong-smelling substance such as disinfectant were accidentally spilled onto a food, it's unlikely that anyone would eat that food. Great care should always be taken to keep cleaning products and disinfectants, which are often kept in the kitchen, well away from food, as well as from children, and in clearly labeled containers. Never transfer household chemicals into food or drink containers, such as empty soda bottles. This common mistake results in many incidents of accidental poisoning of children.

The metals from which many cooking utensils and storage containers are made can be poisonous in the wrong situation, particularly when the item is damaged. Problems usually arise when acidic foods, such as fruit and fruit juice or pickled vegetables, are stored too long in open cans or other metal containers and begin to erode the metal. For example, metal containers used for boiling water have been known to cause poisoning when used to store and dispense fruit juices. In one such incident, a number of school children became ill after drinking orange juice that had been stored in one of these metal pots. The copper in the heating element had dissolved into the acidic fruit juice. Fortunately, the illness was mild and the children recovered.

Potentially Dangerous Metals

Copper in cooking utensils
Antimony in chipped enamelware
Lead and cadmium in glazed pottery
Zinc in galvanized metal containers

SOLID OBJECTS

The solid objects sometimes found in food and drink include pieces of broken machinery and storage containers (resulting from defective equipment) and the bodies of insects, small animals, or birds that have been trapped or fallen into storage containers or processing machinery. Finding such objects is rare, but it can be disturbing when it happens. You can help to prevent this type of contamination from occurring in the home by checking regularly to ensure that storage containers are in good condition and properly sealed and that kitchen equipment is well maintained.

If you find a "foreign body" in a manufactured food, don't just throw it away. Return the product to the place you bought it, or contact the manufacturer—you can usually find a customer service number or address on the packaging. Food manufacturers are usually very concerned about genuine contamination of their products and want to know when things go wrong. They will often want to find the cause of the problem, and if it is widespread, they may recall the product from the stores.

NATURALLY OCCURRING POISONS

Poisons may be naturally present in plants, in many species of mushrooms and other fungi (molds), and in the organs of animals. The symptoms caused by these poisons vary from mild diarrhea to paralysis. Raw haricot beans, for example, contain poisonous chemicals that are destroyed by prolonged boiling, rendering the beans safe to eat. Similarly, the gills of crabs and lobsters contain poisons and should be removed before the shellfish are consumed.

Plants and animals that are normally safe to eat can take up toxic substances from the environment. In some coastal areas, poison-producing plankton species multiply to vast numbers when sea temperatures rise. Filter-feeding shellfish such as clams, oysters, and mussels will accumulate the plankton and its poisons, making the shellfish unsafe to eat. Many of these poisons cause severe symptoms, including diarrhea, paralysis, memory loss, blurred or double vision, and, occasionally, death. Try to ensure that the shellfish you eat are from a reputable source, and if you are gathering them yourself, check with local people that they are safe to harvest.

Environmental pollutants originating from industrial processes, mining, agricultural misuse, and chemical dumping can end up in drinking water or may be taken up by plants and animals. Once these chemicals enter the food chain, they have the potential to poison our food. Concern has been expressed in recent years over the finding of, for example, dioxins and PCBs, both very poisonous to humans, in animals and fish. In one example, thousands of people in northeast England suffered diarrhea in 1984 when their water supply was accidently contaminated with phenolic chemicals.

Food poisoning can also result from eating certain kinds of fish that are not fresh. Poisons are produced as bacteria break down dead flesh. This decomposition releases histamine-like substances, which cause allergic reactions in many people. Eating fish in this state can result in scombrotoxin poisoning, which causes a peppery taste in the mouth, nausea, flushing, and dizziness. Symptoms can start within a few mintues of eating the affected fish, but these usually last only a short time and are rarely fatal. Scombrotoxin poisoning is commonly associated with tuna, albacore, bonito, mahimahi, mackerel, and bluefish, but it is also linked to sardines, pilchards, and herring.

GERMS AND PARASITIC WORMS

The most common causes of food poisoning worldwide are the germs and parasitic worms that can contaminate meat and other foods.

Germs

So-called germs, or microbes, are tiny organisms that can only be seen through a microscope. They exist in vast numbers and are found almost everywhere in the environment. Different types, or species, have been found to withstand extremes of heat, cold, drought, and atmospheric pressure. Although the numbers of different species identified runs into many thousands, only a few hundred normally cause human illness and only a small proportion of these cause food poisoning.

The germs that cause food poisoning fall into three main groups: bacteria, viruses, and protozoa. "Mad cow disease" in humans is related to another agent called a prion. Very little is known about prions and the rare brain-destroying illness they cause (see Chapter 3).

Size of Main Types of Germs			
Type	Example	Relative Size	Visible by
Bacteria	*Salmonella*	1 million on a pinhead	light microscope
Virus	Hepatitis A virus	1 billion on a pinhead	electron microscope
Protozoa	amoeba	5 on a pinhead	human eye (just)

Bacteria

These tiny organisms exist in huge numbers on and in our bodies, but we usually become aware of them only when they make us sick. In fact, the bacteria normally found on or in the body actually help to prevent pathogenic bacteria (those capable of causing disease) from moving in and attacking it. Very few of all the thousands of germs in the environment make people ill, and throughout history, people have found ways of using bacteria and other microbes to their advantage. Probably the best-known use of bacteria is in the making of cheese and yogurt. More recently, scientists have been using bacteria to produce complex chemicals and therapeutic agents, such as insulin, cheaply and in very pure form.

Pathogenic bacteria make us ill by producing poisons (toxins) either in food before we eat it or after contaminated food or drink gets into the digestive system. Some types of pathogenic bacteria pass through the body quickly and cause no long-term illness; others escape from the digestive system and invade other parts of the body, causing serious illness. For example, typhoid fever, which is caused by the bacterium *Salmonella typhi,* is contracted by consuming contaminated food or drink. Once inside the digestive tract, the bacteria penetrate the small intestine and invade the body. Typhoid fever occurs more frequently in underdeveloped regions of the world and is relatively rare in the industrialized countries of western Europe, North America, and Australasia.

The bacteria that most commonly cause food poisoning are listed in the box below. More details about each can be found in the Appendix. For important information about the growth and dangers of bacteria, see the section that begins on page 165.

Common Food-Poisoning Bacteria

Bacillus cereus
Brucella abortus (brucellosis)
Campylobacter (many types)
Clostridium botulinum (botulism)
Clostridium perfringens
Escherichia coli (commonly, *E. coli,* or hamburger disease)
Listeria monocytogenes (listeriosis)
Shigella (several types)
Salmonella typhi and *S. paratyphi* (typhoid)
Salmonella (over 2,000 types causing salmonellosis)
Staphylococcus aureas
Vibrio cholerae (many types, including epidemic cholera)
Vibrio parahaemolyticus
Vibrio vulnificus
Yersinia enterocolitica

Viruses

Viruses are much smaller than bacteria and, unlike bacteria, can multiply only inside living cells. They cannot grow in the food or drink that provides a means of transport for these germs into the body. But once inside, the gastroenteritis-causing viruses invade the tissues of the digestive system, where they hijack cells and then replicate themselves. This causes symptoms of fever, diarrhea, and vomiting, which often start with little warning. The hepatitis A virus targets liver cells, causing yellowing of the skin and eyes known as jaundice (see Appendix).

Most of these viruses are destroyed by the temperatures reached in normal cooking; therefore, virus food poisoning is usually caused by eating either contaminated raw foods or foods that were contaminated after the cooking process. Cooked foods can be contaminated when they are handled by anyone who has viruses on his or her hands. Foods that are eaten raw, such as soft fruit and shellfish, can be a source of the viruses that cause gastroenteritis and jaundice if these foods have been contaminated with sewage. In particular, shellfish such as mussels, clams, and oysters that are harvested from sewage-contaminated coastal waters have been linked to virus gastroenteritis and jaundice.

Protozoa

Foodborne and waterborne protozoa cause illnesses such as cryptosporidiosis and giardiasis.

These single-celled organisms are usually found in watery environments. A few species can cause human illness (see Appendix) and are often associated with poor sanitation. They are generally transmitted by swallowing food or water that has been contaminated with feces. The risk of infection is greatest in regions where standards of sanitation and hygiene are low and where drinking-water quality cannot be guaranteed. In these situations, often found in developing countries, it is wise to take special care over use of water for drinking and ice, brushing teeth, and washing food (see Chapter 17).

The protozoa *Cryptosporidium* and its relatives *Giardia* and *Cyclospora* are now recognized as important causes of diarrhea in both developing and industrialized countries, including the United States. *Cryptosporidium* is particularly tough and can survive not only pasteurization but also the low levels of chlorine often used to make water safe to drink. As a result, outbreaks of illness have occurred in people who drank contaminated pasteurized milk or chlorinated drinking water (see the Appendix for more information).

Parasitic Worms

Infection with parasitic worms is unusual in countries with good meat inspection services but is a definite risk in less-developed regions of the world. Probably the best-known and most common infections are tapeworms and trichinosis. Many parasites go through several stages in their life cycle and may pass through one or more hosts, which may include humans, birds, or animals. Infection occurs when poorly cooked or raw meat containing parasite "cysts" is eaten. Once in the intestine, the cysts develop into worms and cause symptoms. Infection with these parasites is unusual in the United States and Canada and rare in the United Kingdom. Although meat inspection may reduce the risk of infection, the only sure way to be safe is to assume that raw meat could be infected and to ensure that meat is well cooked.

Three types of tapeworm (*Taenia* species) associated with raw or undercooked pork, beef, and freshwater fish cause human illness. Tapeworms have a head with hooks and suckers that attach it to the wall of the intestine. The body is made up of flat segments and may grow to many feet in length. Symptoms of tapeworm infection include abdominal pain and loss of weight, hunger, dizziness, and fatigue because the worm is absorbing the digested food in the intestine.

Trichinosis is associated with eating raw or undercooked meat from a variety of wild animals, including arctic marine mammals, but has been particularly associated with pork and pork products.

Several outbreaks in Europe have been traced to horse meat imported from the United States. Ingested cysts develop into small worms that migrate from the intestine to muscle tissue, causing a variety of symptoms: abdominal and muscle pain, fever, weakness, swelling of the face, pain around the eyes, and conjunctivitis. See the Appendix for more information about trichinosis.

ALLERGIES AND FOOD INTOLERANCE

Common food allergies include intolerance to milk and other dairy products, nuts, wheat products, fish, and seafoods.

Some people react to specific types or classes of foods because they are allergic to the food, intolerant to components of the food, or unable to digest or absorb certain constituents of it. This is not food poisoning as such. The topic of food allergies is beyond the scope of this book, but many excellent books are available on the subject.

GROWTH AND MULTIPLICATION OF BACTERIA

Bacteria multiply by dividing and producing two identical new cells. When conditions are just right, some bacteria, including many of those causing food poisoning, can multiply very rapidly. Doubling in number every twenty minutes, some species of contaminating bacteria quickly reach dangerous levels.

Bacteria can survive, and even multiply, in a wide range of conditions and habitats. Much like humans, food poisoning bacteria need warmth, food, moisture, and time to multiply. But unlike humans, not all bacteria need air.

Warmth

The thermometer shown in the diagram on page 22 is divided into three zones: danger, dead, and dormant. Keeping food out of the danger zone is one of the key rules for safe food handling.

Danger zone

The bacteria that commonly cause food poisoning generally grow and multiply at temperatures between 50°F and 145°F (10°C to 63°C), with an optimum the same as that of the human body—98°F (37°C). Bacterial growth and multiplication begins to slow down when temperatures rise or fall from the ideal range of 70°F to 120°F (21°C to 49°C).

Dead zone

The high temperatures of the dead zone cause increasing damage to the bacterial cells. This damage eventually becomes irreversible, and the cell dies. Even so, the temperature needed to kill cells will vary with the type of bacteria, the length of time it is exposed to high temperatures, and even the food involved. It may take ten minutes or more to kill some bacteria by pasteurization at 163°F (73°C) or by boiling at 212°F (100°C).

To give you an idea of just how tough some bacteria can be, *Bacillus* and *Clostridium* can form heat-resistant spores—special dormant structures that will resist steam at 248°F (120°C) for several minutes. At lower temperatures, these spores grow out, or germinate, to produce cells that may then divide rapidly under the right conditions. It is easy to understand why these bacteria often cause illness when food is warmed up before it is eaten. If a few spores survive the first cooking, they will germinate if the food is then kept at warm temperatures (less than 140°F or 60°C) and will multiply to unsafe levels in a few hours.

Some spores can survive boiling for as long as four hours; some are also unharmed by chemical disinfectants. Therefore, normal

The Effect of Temperature on the Growth of Bacteria

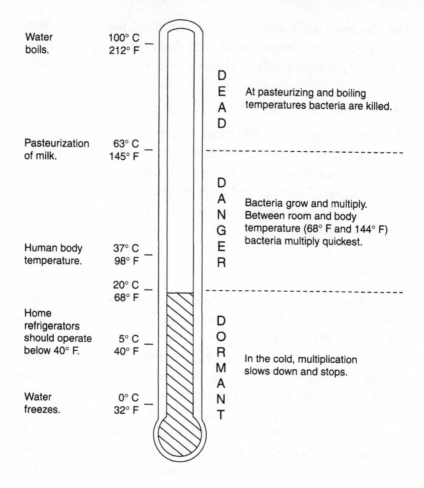

Water boils.	100° C 212° F	
		D E A D — At pasteurizing and boiling temperatures bacteria are killed.
Pasteurization of milk.	63° C 145° F	
		D A N G E R — Bacteria grow and multiply. Between room and body temperature (68° F and 144° F) bacteria multiply quickest.
Human body temperature.	37° C 98° F	
	20° C 68° F	
Home refrigerators should operate below 40° F.	5° C 40° F	D O R M A N T — In the cold, multiplication slows down and stops.
Water freezes.	0° C 32° F	

cooking or disinfecting may not be enough to kill them. They may also survive many years in the environment. When growth conditions become more favorable, spores germinate, grow, and multiply. For example, bacterial spores have been recovered from the wrappings of ancient Egyptian mummies. Having survived in a dormant state for several thousand years, these spores successfully germinated and grew in laboratory experiments.

Dormant zone

At the other end of the scale, bacterial growth and multiplication become progressively slower as the temperature drops into the dormant zone. Most food poisoning bacteria stop growing at domestic refrigerator temperatures of between 35°F and 40°F (2°C and 5°C), but they are still alive.

Some bacteria, including the ones that spoil food and the pathogen *Listeria,* may continue to grow slowly even at refrigerator temperatures. It is difficult to keep a refrigerator at the correct low temperature, and you should check regularly to make sure your refrigerator is running properly. Opening and closing the door frequently, not closing the door completely, and cooling large amounts of warm food, such as a bowl of Jell-O or a beef roast in the refrigerator will raise the temperature inside. Proper use of refrigerators is discussed in detail in Chapter 9.

Food and Moisture

Bacteria, like many other organisms, need food and moisture in order to grow and multiply. And like most organisms, each type of bacteria is specific in its needs.

Danger foods

The foods that best support bacterial growth include those with a lot of protein and moisture, such as meat. *Salmonella* are more likely to be found in raw foods such as meat, poultry, and eggs, whereas *Clostridium* prefer cooked and reheated foods such as stews and gravies. *Staphylococci,* which often originate on human skin, are commonly spread by a food preparer who has handled the food and then left it at room temperature for a while before consumption. *Bacillus* and its spores survive on grains and cereals, ready to spring to life in the right conditions.

Foods Associated with *Salmonella* Infection

Meat and poultry
Eggs and dairy products
Fermented salami sausage snacks
Infant milk formulas
Melons
Bean sprouts
Corn-based snacks
Dried peppercorns and other spices
Chocolate
Tea leaves

Although dried foods such as infant formula and powdered milk, eggs, and soups do not contain enough moisture to allow bacteria to grow, these products are not necessarily free of bacteria and dormant spores. As soon as the product is reconstituted by adding water, there is a possibility that any bacteria present will revive and begin to grow and multiply. To avoid problems with reconstituted dried foods, follow these four simple rules:

1. If possible, consume the food immediately after reconstituting it.
2. Only make up what you can use immediately, thus avoiding the need to store the food.
3. Keep reconstituted food out of the danger zone by keeping it piping hot if you are going to eat it soon; if you cannot eat it right away, refrigerate it as soon as it is cool.
4. Always keep the food covered.

Time Bombs

Given the right combination of food, moisture, and a temperature around 98°F (37°C), bacteria can divide very rapidly.

Given enough time, just a few bacteria can multiply to dangerous levels.

Imagine what could happen if a piece of meat containing a thousand bacteria were left at room temperature for just four hours. In just three hours and twenty minutes, there will be 1 million bacteria present. By the time four hours have passed, the numbers will have increased to over 4 million. It takes very little imagination to realize what will be happening on a fresh chicken left with the groceries in a car trunk for a couple of hours on a warm summer day. Research shows that a large proportion of chickens are contaminated with food poisoning bacteria. By the time that chicken reaches the kitchen, it has become a potential biological time bomb capable of leaving large numbers of bacteria on any surface it touches—including your hands.

> FOOD SHOULD NOT BE LEFT IN THE TEMPERATURE DANGER ZONE FOR MORE THAN A TOTAL OF TWO HOURS.

Anaerobic Bacteria

Bacteria that need air for growth are called aerobes. Bacteria that live in the absence of oxygen are called anaerobes. Probably the best-known of the anaerobic food poisoning bacteria is *Clostridium botulinum,* which causes botulism. If this bacteria gets into a canned or bottled food and is able to multiply, it produces a deadly poison that causes an unusual but very serious type of food poisoning that requires prompt medical treatment. See the Appendix for more about botulism. The potential dangers of home bottling and canning are described in Chapter 13.

3

EGGS, HAMBURGERS, BERRIES, WATER, AND MAD COW DISEASE

SALMONELLA

The *Salmonella* bacterium has been linked to a wide variety of foods, particularly poultry and other meats. Occasional problems due to *Salmonella*-contaminated eggs had been noted for many years, but during the mid-1980s, public health scientists in the United States and the United Kingdom began receiving increasing numbers of reports suggesting that chicken eggs were causing food poisoning. Investigations confirmed that these recent outbreaks were the result of *Salmonella* bacteria being passed from infected egg-laying chickens to the inside of the egg. This makes contamination difficult to detect but easy to pass on. Here's the current situation:

- Human infections are linked to eggs contaminated on the inside, not on the outside; therefore, care in handling the egg will not reduce the possibility of infection. Protection from infection relies on cooking the egg well.
- This problem has led to rapid and, in some countries, dramatic increases in human infection caused by strains (variants) of one *Salmonella*—*S. enteritidis.*

26

- Since first appearing in the mid-1980s, egg-associated *Salmonella enteritidis* infection has occurred virtually worldwide.

Human *Salmonella* infection specifically linked to eating raw or undercooked eggs is now recognized as an important public health issue in many countries. Considerable efforts are being made to understand and control this problem, but at present, people at higher risk—that is, the very young and the elderly as well as individuals with depressed immune systems caused by existing serious illness, AIDS, immunity-suppressing treatments such as chemotherapy and radiotherapy, or pregnancy—should eat only well-cooked eggs and should avoid raw and undercooked eggs altogether.

HAMBURGER DISEASE: *E. COLI*

In the early 1980s, outbreaks of food poisoning caused by the bacteria *Escherichia coli*, commonly called *E. coli*, were linked to eating undercooked hamburgers. So, "hamburger disease" was added to the list of causes of food poisoning. In its severest form, symptoms included bloody diarrhea and progressed to temporary or permanent kidney failure and death. Young children, particularly those under age five, were at greatest risk of having a severe illness.

The disease is caused by strains of the *E. coli* that make verotoxins. Although one particular strain, *E. coli* O157, is the most common cause of this disease, other strains can also produce these poisons.

Cattle appear to harbor these bacteria, so it is not surprising that beef and, especially, undercooked ground beef products such as hamburgers, are a major source of this type of food poisoning. Milk and dairy products as well as water have also been identified as the source of infection in some outbreaks. *E. coli* can also be spread from one person to another, and one outbreak was linked to swimming in a lake used by a large number of people.

Protective measures against *E. coli* include maintaining high standards of hygiene in the kitchen to limit spread of the germ and, most important, ensuring that hamburgers are cooked thoroughly until there is no sign of any pink or red meat. If you are served a hamburger that is still red or pink in the middle, don't hesitate to send it back for more cooking.

DIARRHEA AND BERRIES

Since 1995, several outbreaks of diarrhea in the United States and Canada have been traced to eating soft fruits, such as raspberries. The culprit is a parasite called *Cyclospora*. Infection with this tiny, single-celled, protozoa-like parasite leads to diarrhea, abdominal pain, fever, vomiting, nausea, and fatigue. Symptoms can last from a few days to over a month if not treated, and they may last many months in people with depressed immunity.

Studies of *Cyclospora* are incomplete, but it seems that the parasite is transmitted in contaminated water, particularly in developing countries. Contamination of soft fruit, largely from South America, may have been the result of irrigating fields with contaminated water or of contact with the contaminated hands of fruit pickers or handlers during harvesting and processing.

Thorough washing of fruit with clean water will reduce the chances of infection but may not remove all the parasites. High temperatures and freezing may be effective in killing *Cyclospora*.

WATERY PROBLEMS

Most people in modern developed countries tend to think that they are well protected against waterborne illness, particularly waterborne gastroenteritis. But in recent years, there have been a number of outbreaks in both North America and Europe of a waterborne parasite called *Cryptosporidium*. Of greatest concern has been the infection of communities receiving municipal, treated water supplies. So what has gone wrong?

Cryptosporidium is a protozoa-like parasite found in a number of domestic and wild animals as well as in humans, and its excretion by animals may lead to contamination of the environment, including water sources. Unfortunately, *Cryptosporidium* is resistant to chlorine used to purify drinking water, and unless infected water is filtered, it will remain a potential source of infection to anyone drinking it. Infection in healthy people results in a diarrhea illness that may come and go for up to a month. In people with depressed immunity, especially those with AIDS, the infection is usually chronic and can lead to death.

"Crypto" An outbreak of *Cryptosporidium* in Milwaukee infected more than 400,000 people and left 104 people dead. The source of this outbreak—drinking water.

MAD COW DISEASE

This new disease, whose scientific name is bovine spongiform encephalopathy, or BSE, first appeared in 1985 in England, where it spread rapidly in cattle herds. In the infected animal, the disease causes changes in behavior, weakness, lack of coordination, and finally death. These symptoms are caused by damage to the animal's brain, which eventually has so many holes in it that when viewed through a microscope, it looks like a sponge.

BSE is only one of a number of similar diseases that have been found in several types of animals as well as in humans. These include scrapie in sheep, mad squirrel disease, and Creutzfeldt-Jakob disease, or CJD, in humans. Not much is known about these diseases except that they are caused by agents called prions, which in some situations, can be passed around. It is known that prions can survive normal cooking, freezing, and irradiation.

British cattle are thought to have been infected by feed made from sheep remains contaminated by the scrapie agent. This probably followed changes in the way the feed products were produced, including lower processing temperatures and a reduction in the amounts of solvents used. Laboratory experiments have shown that the BSE agent can infect other animals. Controls introduced by the British government since 1988 have included slaughter of infected or exposed cattle and a ban on the use of some offal, particularly the brain and the spinal cord, in animal feeds. There has been a big reduction in BSE-infected cattle in Britain in the last few years, but a similar disease has been found in small numbers of cattle in other countries.

Fears have been expressed about the possibility that BSE, which probably came from scrapie-infected sheep, might also infect humans and cause a CJD-like illness. Although this was first thought to be unlikely, a number of cases of a new type, or variant, of CJD has been reported in Britain since 1996.

Although CJD occurs worldwide, affecting about one person in 1 million each year, it is more common in some family clusters reported in Slovakia, Israel, and Chile, and it usually occurs in people over age forty. The "new" CJD cases, however, have slightly different symptoms, have no obvious ethnic or family associations, and have occurred in a number of younger people.

At the end of 1997, more than twenty cases of this new variant CJD had been reported in Britain. Recent evidence strongly suggests that the prion causing BSE in cattle is the same as the one causing the new variant CJD in people—and that cases in Britain are linked to eating contaminated beef. It is still not clear whether the new CJD cases in Britain are the start of an epidemic. The incubation period of this disease may last several years, and it will be some time before public health authorities can accurately measure the real risk.

How widespread is the risk?

Although a handful of new CJD cases have been reported in other European countries where there were infected cattle, there is no evidence of an increased risk of infection in the United States or in Canada. British cattle, because of the very strict regulations imposed on its production, is probably now a safe source of beef.

ANTIBIOTIC RESISTANCE AND FOOD POISONING GERMS

Public health authorities in the United States, Canada, and the United Kingdom have been monitoring an increase in human and animal infection with a new strain of *Salmonella typhimurium,* a bacterium that has been found in cattle and humans for many years. This new strain, known as phage type 104, is resistant to a wide range of common antibiotics, including ampicillin, chloramphenicol, ciprofloxacin, streptomycin, sulfonamides, tetracycline, and trimethoprim. Resistance basically means that the germ is able to survive attack by normal treatment doses of the antibiotic. Because this new strain is able to resist these antibiotics, it would be difficult to treat if it escaped from the intestines of an infected person and invaded other parts of the body.

The number of human cases of the new strain began to rise rapidly from a few hundred in 1990 in the United Kingdom to about four thousand cases in 1996. This rise in human cases followed an earlier increase in infections in cattle. The number of human cases of this *Salmonella* in North America have also risen over the last two years.

So where did this very resistant *Salmonella* come from? Its appearance and spread first in cattle suggests that its origins are linked to this sector of the agricultural industry. A number of reports in Europe and North America going back as far as 1968 have suggested that the use of antibiotics in the animal industry could lead to the appearance of resistant bacteria. The truth may not be quite so simple.

How Does Antibiotic Resistance Develop?

Antibiotics for treating bacterial infection have been around since penicillin and sulfonamides became available before the 1940s. Antibiotics work by interfering with the growth or multiplication of the bacterial cell. These special chemicals fall into families, or groups, depending on how they work or whether they are chemically similar. Some bacteria are naturally able to resist antibiotics; others develop resistance by "learning" to prevent the antibiotic from working effectively. This may happen when bacteria are continuously exposed to an antibiotic at a low level that allows spontaneous mutants to appear—mutants that have built-in resistance. Alternatively, bacteria may share bits of genetic information (DNA) that already carry instructions giving resistance to antibiotics.

The presence of antibiotics in animals and in the environment may encourage the development of resistant bacteria. Antibiotics get into the environment in a number of ways.

Agricultural Use:
- Large quantities of antibiotics have, for many years, been used by the agricultural industry for treating animal diseases, as a feed additive to prevent disease or at low levels as a growth promoter. In 1985 an estimated 9.5 million kilograms of antibiotics were given to cattle, pigs, and poultry in the United States; 7.3 million kilograms, used at levels below that needed to fight infection, were given as a preventive measure or to promote animal growth. Only 1.1 million kilograms (13 percent) was given for actually treating sick animals. While more recent estimates were not available, United States government experts were reported in 1995 to

assert that the use of antibiotics in agriculture is declining. However, without current, detailed information on the types and quantities of antibiotics being used in agriculture and the reasons for their use, it is difficult to assess actual trends.

- Antibiotics are sprayed on plants and vegetables to prevent growth of plant pathogens.
- Commercial fish farming uses antibiotics to treat or prevent fish disease. This is done either through the use of medicated feed or by direct spraying.

Medical Use:
- Antibiotics are one of the most commonly prescribed medicines. They are excreted by the body and eventually end up in the environment.
- Antibiotics are overused in human medicine and are sometimes given for illnesses for which they are not effective, for example, colds and influenza.

The presence of antibiotics in the environment, through their widespread use in agriculture, aquaculture, and human medicine, increases evolutionary pressures that select the microbes that prove able to survive.

PART TWO

FOOD POISONING
AND YOU

4

SYMPTOMS
AND COMPLICATIONS
OF FOOD POISONING

This book uses the term "food poisoning" in a general way to describe the illnesses caused by the germs that can attack people through food. The actual symptoms of food poisoning can vary widely, depending on the type of germ causing the illness and the way in which it makes people ill (see Chapter 18). Most people who get food poisoning experience the diarrhea and vomiting normally associated with gastrointestinal upsets, but others develop rarer and more serious complications.

COMMON SYMPTOMS AND THEIR SEVERITY

Most people think of food poisoning as an illness that usually causes diarrhea or vomiting, or both. These are certainly the most common and most easily recognized symptoms, but food poisoning can appear in many disguises. Symptoms vary depending on the germ or the poison it produces, on where in the body the attack takes place, and on the health of the victim. An attack on the digestive passage, for example, will probably include combinations of the following symptoms:

Diarrhea, sometimes with blood, mucus, or bile present

Nausea (feeling sick)

Vomiting (being sick)

Headache

Fever (high temperatures usually accompanied by sweats and chills)

Stomach pains and/or cramps

Dizziness

Stomach Flu

People who are suffering from a combination of common symptoms of gastrointestinal upset often complain of having "stomach flu." In fact, there is no such thing as stomach flu. Flu is a respiratory illness caused by the flu virus. What they are most likely experiencing is an attack of food poisoning.

Any of these symptoms can range from mild to very severe, but in healthy people, these symptoms will usually subside within one to five days. So for most healthy teenagers and adults, the symptoms are rarely more than an unpleasant inconvenience that goes away with time, rest, and intake of plenty of fluids. But if the symptoms seem unusually severe or if they persist, seek medical advice.

The common symptoms caused by a range of specific germs are described in the Appendix.

The Very Young and the Elderly

For infants, young children, and the elderly, symptoms such as vomiting, diarrhea, and fever can be dangerous, and it is always wise to seek medical advice if symptoms persist for more than twenty-four hours. The physical acts of vomiting and diarrhea can cause damage, such as tearing, to delicate or weakened internal tissues. Frequent, prolonged diarrhea and vomiting can rapidly cause dehydration, with potentially serious results—especially in babies less than a year old. The body of a young child is not fully equipped to deal with fevers, which may result in seizures. Fanning and sponging the child's body with tepid water can help bring down the temperature and reduce the risk of convulsion, but medical advice should be sought as soon as possible.

The Dangers of Dehydration

Dehydration occurs when the body loses excessive amounts of body fluids and chemicals called electrolytes, principally sodium and potassium. This loss can be very serious and can occur rapidly with severe diarrhea and vomiting, particularly in babies and young children. Fluids can be replaced by oral rehydration (OR)—giving fluids containing the right balance of electrolytes by mouth.

Pharmacists usually stock packets of OR electrolytes, which can be added to cooled, boiled water and given to the sick person. It is a wise precaution to take some of these packets on vacation, especially when visiting underdeveloped countries. Seek medical advice for young children and adults with prolonged symptoms. Patients with severe dehydration may be admitted to a hospital and put on an intravenous drip, which rapidly replaces fluids and electrolytes lost when diarrhea and vomiting persist.

COMPLICATIONS OF FOOD POISONING

When a microbe or its toxin penetrates the digestive tract and invades other parts of the body, a wide variety of symptoms can result, depending on which organ(s) (e.g., brain, kidney, liver) or system (e.g., circulatory system, nervous system) is affected. For example, the toxin produced by the bacteria *Clostridium botulinum*, which causes botulism, heads for the nervous system, causing symptoms such as double vision, giddiness, nausea, headache, and, if untreated, eventual paralysis and death. The hepatitis A virus aims for the liver, where it affects liver function and results in jaundice. *Trichinella spiralis*, the parasitic worm that causes trichinosis, settles in muscles, causing muscle pains and pain around the eyes. The bacteria *Salmonella typhi*, which causes typhoid, invades the circulatory system and the spleen, causing prolonged fever and, if untreated, multiple complications and death.

Here are some other complications that can occur following food poisoning:

Blood poisoning (septicemia)
Swelling of the tissues around the heart and damage to the
    heart valves and blood vessels
Swelling of the brain tissue (meningitis)
Damage to bones and joints, including a type of arthritis
Damage to kidneys and liver and other vital organs
Paralysis
Pneumonia
Abortion
Damaged brain function (e.g., memory loss)

Fortunately, these complications are fairly unusual, and many will resolve with prompt treatment. Research suggests that two to three of every hundred food poisoning cases develop long-term illnesses. Some of these long-term illnesses may last for months; others will become lifelong problems.

Arthritis

Prolonged disability from reactive arthritis following diarrhea illness caused by *Salmonella, Shigella, Campylobacter,* and *Yersinia* infection may affect as many as two hundred thousand people each year in the United States alone. Research indicates that some individuals may be genetically more likely to develop this condition.

Hemolytic Uremic Syndrome (HUS)

This is one of the devastating complications that follow the *E. coli* infection known as hamburger disease. HUS causes kidney failure, and although some patients recover, others need long-term kidney dialysis or a transplant, and some die. It has been estimated that as many as twenty thousand people get hamburger disease each year in the United States, many of them young children. About three in every thousand will develop the long-term effects.

Abortion and Congenital Illness

Complications associated with food poisoning can affect unborn babies in two ways: death of the fetus or permanant impairment of the baby. For example, infection of the mother with the parasite *Toxoplasma* in early pregnancy can lead to the death of the fetus or result in serious disorders including brain damage, visual impairment, hearing loss, hydrocephaly, microcephaly, and liver problems. Infection of the mother in late pregnancy can result in only mild or symptomless infection of the unborn baby, followed by delayed affects such as chronic visual problems.

Guillain-Barré Syndrome

This type of acute paralysis has been associated with *Campylobacter* infection. Although 70 to 80 percent of patients recover over a period of weeks or months, a small proportion are permanently disabled and some die. Patients may need to have their breathing assisted by a ventilator, and they can experience weeks or months of severe pain.

Food Poisoning and Loss of Memory

In 1987, an outbreak of food poisoning in Canada caused by demoic acid resulted from eating shellfish harvested from coastal areas containing high levels of a particular type of algae. Many of those affected experienced loss of memory.

WHO GETS FOOD POISONING?

Practical advice on safe cooking for those with special needs is given in Part Five.

Anyone can get food poisoning, but three main factors strongly influence whether a person becomes ill and whether the illness becomes severe: health, life-style, and nutrition and diet.

Health

Your overall health plays a critical role in whether you will get infections. Larger doses of germs are needed to cause illness in young healthy adults than are needed in other segments of the general population. Here are the groups that are most at risk of getting ill:

Children under age five and adults over sixty-five
People with depressed immune systems
Individuals with existing medical conditions

The number of people in these higher-risk groups is growing each year in most industrialized countries. In the United States, this is currently about 25 percent of the population and the numbers are increasing. In the early 1990s, these were the major higher-risk populations in the United States:

Seniors over age sixty-five	29.4 million
Pregnant women	5.7 million
Babies under four weeks old	4.0 million
Cancer patients	2.4 million
Transplant patients	0.1 million
AIDS patients	0.1 million

The biggest group, people over sixty-five, is increasing by about 1 million every year. For each higher-risk group, the major problem is a loss of the body's ability to fight infections—a loss of immunity. For some, this may be "natural," in the sense that it occurs as a result of pregnancy or as part of the aging process or because it is linked to inherited factors. For others, loss of immunity results from outside causes, which can include the following:

Infection (AIDS)
Preexisting medical conditions
Chemotherapy and radiation treatments
Lifestyle factors
Nutrition

Pregnancy

A woman's immune system is suppressed during pregnancy. This temporary change is designed to protect the developing fetus from attack by the mother's immune system, and it has only a slight effect on her ability to fight infection. However, there is evidence that pregnant women are more vulnerable to viruses and to bacteria such as *Listeria*.

Age

Babies are born with an immature immune system, which matures during the first two years of life; and during this time, they are more open to infection. Up to age five, children are at a higher risk because their small body weight needs only a very small dose of germs to make them ill. At the other end of the age spectrum, the body's ability to fight infection begins to decline from about age forty-five. The end result is that the elderly are unable to fight a long battle against infection. In addition, the secretion of stomach acids decreases with age, and this allows bacteria an easier passage to the intestines.

Inherited factors

Some individuals may inherit either a decreased ability to fight disease or factors that make them more likely to develop long-term complications. For example, sickle cell disease, an inherited disorder that occurs mainly in people of African or Caribbean descent, damages the blood system and makes the body more vulnerable to infection. Affected individuals are thus more likely to develop complications after infections with germs such as *Salmonella.*

Infection

Some infections can decrease a person's ability to resist attack by another germ. Individuals with AIDS, for example, die not from the HIV virus that causes AIDS, but from infections or other medical conditions that arise because the HIV virus has severely damaged the immune system. People with AIDS are therefore very vulnerable to infections, including those caused by germs found in food and water, such as *Salmonella* and *Cryptosporidium.* In AIDS patients, *Cryptosporidium* is a common cause of diarrhea, and the infection is usually chronic.

At present, over 230,000 people in the United States have AIDS, and an estimated 600,000 are infected with the HIV virus.

These people and their caregivers need to give special attention to the safe preparation of food.

Preexisting medical conditions

Any preexisting illness may increase the likelihood or severity of food poisoning, either because the illness is affecting the body's ability to fight infection or because treatment is damaging the body's defense systems. Patients with leukemia, for example, are vulnerable because their white blood cells, which normally fight infection, are damaged or immature and are therefore unable to do their job. In addition, certain organs, such as the spleen, play important roles in the body's defense system, especially in fighting infections caused by bacteria. Removal of the spleen as a result of disease or injury would therefore have a big impact on the body's ability to resist bacteria. Any condition that requires removal of part of the stomach reduces acid production and increases the possibility that germs in food will reach the intestines.

Chemotherapy and radiation therapy

Deliberate suppression of the immune system is common in the treatment of a wide variety of conditions, including rheumatoid arthritis, cancers, and organ transplants. People undergoing such treatment are very susceptible to infection by germs, including some commonly found in food but which pose little threat to healthy individuals. The number of such at-risk individuals increase every year, and in the United States, the number of transplant patients alone are increasing by 50 percent each year.

Lifestyle

The link between the stresses of life and the body's ability to resist infection is just beginning to be understood. Research has shown that persistent stress, which can be caused by a wide range of factors—from loneliness to chronic illness or pain, to dangerous environmental factors, to a poor ability to cope—decreases the efficiency of the immune system. The result is that attacking germs can get established more easily or that fewer germs are needed to cause illness.

Both smoking and alcoholism seem to put people at a higher risk for food poisoning. Smoking affects the immune system, and alcoholism leads to a reduction in liver and kidney function. This causes an increase of iron in the blood, which can in turn, encourage the growth of some bacteria found in food and water.

Nutrition and Diet

The tissues in the body that produce white blood cells and other infection-fighting factors have a very high energy demand and are very sensitive to a lack or an excess of many nutrients. Therefore, insufficient protein, carbohydrates, and certain vitamins (A, B, C, folic acid) and minerals (zinc and iron) as well as too much cholesterol and fat affect the ability of the immune system to work effectively. Here are the most common reasons for inadequate intake of essential nutrients, or malnutrition:

Food just not being available, as in situations of poverty or famine.
Poor food choices, or use of poor-quality ingredients.
Medical conditions that interfere with the way in which the body takes in nutrients, usually in ill or elderly persons.

Unfortunately, malnutrition often occurs in situations where people are also at high risk of infection by foodborne and waterborne germs resulting from poor sanitation and hygiene. These include the obvious situations of famine centers and refugee camps, areas of economic disaster, inner cities, and even residential facilities caring for incontinent patients.

In addition to the risks of malnutrition, food or drink can affect the risk of getting food poisoning in several ways. The most obvious way is through ingestion of contaminated food. Some foods do seem to be more likely to be contaminated with germs (see Chapter 7). For example, as many as thirty to eighty of every hundred chickens on sale in the supermarket may be contaminated with *Salmonella* or *Campylobacter* or both. Raw shellfish harvested from water contaminated by sewage often harbors a variety of human pathogens, including bacteria and viruses. These and similar foods can cause illness, either when they are not cooked well enough to kill the germs, or when their handling and preparation causes other foods to become contaminated, known as cross-contamination. Advice on prevention of cross-contamination when shopping is given in Part Three; ways to prevent cross-contamination in the kitchen are given in Part Four.

5

WHAT TO DO IF YOU GET FOOD POISONING

Most food poisoning occurs in the home, but it is also commonly linked to other settings, including restaurants, snack bars, various institutions, schools, and large social gatherings, such as receptions.

It is always hoped that food preparers in any situation will take precautions to ensure that they are providing food that is safe to eat. If you have symptoms of diarrhea or vomiting, DO NOT prepare food for other people if at all possible. If you really must prepare food, take extra care with washing your hands, especially after using the toilet and always before you touch food. Also, choose foods that will be well cooked and will be eaten right away.

But inevitably, mistakes are made and some people become ill. If you suspect that you or a member of your family has food poisoning, here are a few simple suggestions about what to do.

Coping with Mild Symptoms

If your symptoms are mild, you can probably treat yourself. Even if you don't feel like eating, it is important to keep up your intake of fluids. Rest and drink plenty of cooled, boiled water, apple juice, or tea. Drink oral rehydration fluid if you have it. Drinking plenty of fluids helps you to replace those lost through diarrhea, vomiting, and sweating.

Treating Severe Symptoms and High-Risk People

If symptoms are severe and continue for more than a few hours, or if the ill person is a baby, an elderly person, or someone who falls into one of the higher-risk groups described in the box below, seek medical advice as soon as possible. Either consult your physician or go to the nearest hospital emergency room. (For more details about higher-risk groups, see Chapter 4.)

Seek Medical Advice Immediately for These High-Risk Groups

Infants and young children
Elderly people
Pregnant women
People with AIDS
People with existing serious illness
People taking treatments that depress immunity (e.g., chemotherapy)

Reporting the Illness

When to report

If you think that your illness was caused by a commercial product bought at a particular store or by something you ate at a large gathering or a public eating place, you should report it to your local or regional public health office. (You'll find the number listed under state offices in the white pages of your phone directory. Your town hall or local police department should also have a contact telephone number.) By reporting the incident, you might be helping to prevent others from becoming ill.

What to report

When you make your report, try to have the following information ready:

> Your name, address, and telephone number
> Where the suspect food was eaten, *or*
> The name of the suspect product and where it was bought
> When the food was eaten and when you became ill
> Reports of or names of any others who became ill after eating
>   the same meal

If you suspect a commercial product, have the container available if possible. This has important information on it, including a *lot* or *batch* number that will help public health officials trace its source, as well as the manufacturer's name and address. If you still have the suspect food, seal it in a plastic bag and put it in the refrigerator and label DO NOT USE. Tell the person to whom you make the report that you have the suspect food, and ask if it will be wanted for laboratory tests. If so, the public health office should arrange to collect the item. If not, ask for advice on how to safely dispose of it.

Finally, you may be asked to cooperate in a wider investigation. This usually happens when public health officials suspect that a lot of people have been affected or that the contaminated food is widespread. Taking part in these investigations can help to rapidly identify an important cause of food poisoning, and it may help prevent others from getting sick.

PART THREE

HOW TO PREVENT FOOD POISONING WHEN SHOPPING

6

CHOOSING WHERE TO SHOP FOR FOOD

> **Golden Rule:** Look out for visual clues, and follow your instincts.

Safe food handling begins at the store where you select and purchase your food. From that point on, what happens to the food is largely determined by you. It's not difficult to shop safely; it's just a question of paying attention to the visual clues around you and listening to your instincts.

VISUAL CLUES FOR A SAFE FOOD STORE

First, be aware of the store itself. It should look clean and well maintained, and there should be no rotting food left around, either inside the store or outside around the trash area. The store should be free from flies and other insects and, of course, rodents. Except for guide dogs, all pets should be kept out of food stores. Stores should be brightly lighted so that you can clearly see what you are buying. Stores located in hot climates should be air conditioned. All food (except for anything in glass, cans, or wrapped in heavy plastic) should be kept at least 6 inches off the floor.

In much the same way that you look at the store itself, look at the people who work there. They should be clean and tidy in appearance and be wearing clean clothes. In areas of the store such as the deli counter, the meat department, and the bakery, employees may be required to wear a hat and disposable gloves as well as aprons in order to protect the food from contamination. Food staff should not have open wounds, sores, or even a bad case of acne. All wounds should be covered with clean dressings. The law prohibits smoking in a food store, although local regulations may vary for small stores that double as lunch or breakfast stands.

Shopping from Market Stalls and Farm Stands

In many parts of the United States and around the world, fresh produce and other foods can be purchased from market traders, local farmer's markets, and farm stands. Produce that comes direct from local farms is often fresher, tastier, and cheaper than store-bought produce. But the advice for safe food shopping is the same wherever you buy the food. Meat, poultry, and seafood should be purchased only from stalls with refrigeration units and where the food is protected from contamination by flies, animals, and passers-by. Foods like milk, eggs, cheese, yogurt, bacon, and ham should also be purchased only from refrigerated stalls where they are protected from contamination. Home-baked pies and cakes should be wrapped and protected from contamination. Some farms may even sell unpasteurized milk direct to the public, but there is always a risk of food poisoning from drinking untreated milk, and it is not recommended by food safety experts.

HOW TO BECOME A REVOLTING CONSUMER

One of the first lessons about food safety is that we all need to become more proactive, so that we can protect both ourselves and others. Shopping for groceries can be a time-consuming and tedious chore, but simply incorporating the advice given in the following chapters into your shopping routine can help you to avoid many problems. To be a safe shopper, you may also have to become a Revolting Consumer. If you are unhappy about conditions at your store, the most effective way to get things changed is to speak up and speak out. If you see something that seems wrong—some rotting produce, or a clerk in a dirty apron, or some packaged sliced ham that has passed its sell-by date, for example—don't just make a mental note to call the local food inspector when you get home or quietly decide not to shop there again. *Call for the manager.* Tell him or her politely but loudly just what it is that you are concerned about, and unless you have just come across the sloppiest store manager in the state, you will get a positive response and some fast remedial action. A good store manager will not risk the possible loss of business that your loud complaint may cause when the other customers hear you. If by chance you do run into the sloppiest store manager, then by all means call the food inspector at your local public health office and make a note not to shop at the store again until things improve.

Inspections of Food Stores

Both federal and state food and sanitary codes require regular inspections of all food establishments in the United States. In addition to looking for safe food practice and sanitary conditions, the codes allow the flexibility to respond to new issues as they occur. Some states require twice-yearly inspections and more if necessary. Others require mandated training of managers and other personnel. In Great Britain, all food businesses must register with the local authority, and the law has recently gotten tougher. Stores are now given a priority rating based on factors that include what type of food is sold, whether the store sells to high-risk groups such as a nursing home, and general confidence in the management's abilities. The rating determines the frequency of inspection. For example, these days, butcher's shops may find themselves inspected every six months instead of the previous annual inspection.

7

SHOPPING FOR FOOD

SELECTING FRESH MEAT

Meat and poultry are the major food source of food poisoning germs in both domestic and commercial kitchens. United States Department of Agriculture (USDA) estimates in 1993 showed that most food poisoning came from eating contaminated meat or poultry, including 50 to 75 percent of *Salmonella* infections, 75 percent of *Campylobacter* infections, and 75 percent of *E. coli* O157 infections. Many of these germs are naturally occurring contaminants of animal digestive systems, so this is not a new problem; but the problem does seem to have gotten worse over the last decade. Intensification of agribusiness and the animal slaughter process are both likely contributory factors. It only takes one contaminated chicken in the processing line to cause contamination of many other birds that may then be distributed for sale around the country.

> **Golden Rule:** Switch into "alert mode." Check for sell-by dates, smell, color, and leaky packaging.

Most stores offer you a choice in buying fresh meat: You can choose pre-wrapped, weighed, and priced packages of meat from refrigerated shelves, or you can select cuts from a refrigerated meat counter and have them weighed, wrapped, and priced by a meat clerk. Only buy meat that has been kept cool (or frozen) at less than 40°F (5°C)—there should be a thermometer visible along the shelves. Whatever way you choose to buy meat, you really need to switch into "alert mode" at this point. You cannot detect the presence of germs on the meat, but here are a few things to watch out for.

Date stamps

If buying prepackaged meat, first look for the date stamp. Always buy within the sell-by or best-before date (these terms differ by country). Purchase ground beef only on the day that it is ground.

Leaky packaging

Cuts of meat and meat products are usually placed on polyfoam trays and covered with clear plastic food wrap. The packaging often leaks meat juices, and it is important to remember that these juices are likely to be contaminated—you should avoid getting them onto your hands or onto other foods in your cart. If the meat is not well wrapped, then call a meat clerk and ask for the package to be re-wrapped. If you do get meat juices on your hands, then ask the clerk for some antibacterial handiwipes. Place prepackaged meats in plastic bags from the fruit-and-vegetable section for added protection.

Odor and color

Use your senses of smell and sight. Don't purchase any meat that has an unpleasant odor. Cuts of beef should be bright cherry red color, and although the outer surfaces of ground beef and steaks are often brown in color, the inside should be pink to red. Lamb should be light red, and pork should look pink with white fat and have a firm texture. Reject any meat that is brown or greenish in color; that has brown, green, or purple blotches or black, white, or green spots; or that has a slimy or sticky texture. Poultry should have no discoloration and should have a firm texture and no stickiness under wings and around joints. Bad odor and discoloration on meat and poultry are signs that the food is spoiling, either because it is not fresh or because it has been badly handled, badly packaged, or badly stored. The signs do not indicate the presence of food poisoning germs, but they certainly do indicate that things are going wrong and that the food should be avoided.

Meat and poultry stamps

It's also a good idea to look for meat and poultry stamps. You may see a stamp showing that the meat or poultry has been inspected by the USDA or by a state department of health. The USDA can also grade meat and poultry. This stamp identifies the relative quality of the meat.

Organic Meat

People often ask whether meat from organically raised animals is less likely to be contaminated with food poisoning germs than is meat from traditionally raised animals. The answer is that there is not enough information available to make valid comparisons. Many food poisoning germs are naturally present in animals' digestive systems, and there is no reason to believe that these germs will not be present in organically raised animals. On the other hand, organically raised animals are usually less intensively raised and may be less stressed and less prone to infection. Unfortunately, even if the animals are raised in less contaminated conditions, once they are sent to slaughter along with animals from all other sources, then there is little control on cross-contamination between carcasses.

A customer at an organic meat counter once asked if the beef was free of *E. coli* O157, because he liked to eat his beef cooked rare. The meat clerk replied that the animals were monitored for

E. coli up to their entry to the slaughterhouse. The customer took this to mean that the meat was indeed *E. coli*–free and was satisfied with this answer. In fact, there is no way that the meat clerk could know the *E. coli* status of the meat if it was not sampled after slaughter.

SELECTING FRESH SEAFOOD

Here, again, you need to use good judgment and select carefully. Fish, shellfish, and crabs living in water contaminated by sewage often contain the bacteria and virus germs that can cause food poisoning. Because shellfish feed by filtering water, they concentrate any germs from polluted waters within their own bodies. Shellfish are often the cause of viral food poisoning, probably because they are frequently eaten raw or are cooked less thoroughly than other seafood.

Seafood Toxins

The risks of illness from seafood toxins cannot be predicted from the appearance of the fish. If you have any concerns, ask the fish clerk or the store manager for information about the source of the fish or shellfish. All shellfish should come from licensed commercial beds.

Fresh fish, shellfish (clams, mussels, and oysters), and crustacea (lobsters, crab, and shrimp) should be displayed at cool temperatures less than 40°F (5°C). Seafood is highly perishable and is usually on display packed with ice in order to keep it as fresh as possible. Clerks at seafood counters wear plastic gloves in order to avoid causing any contamination themselves.

> **Golden Rule:** Fresh fish does not smell *fishy*.

Fresh fish does not have a fishy odor; the eyes are bright, clear, and full; and the texture of the flesh and belly are firm. The shells of shellfish should be closed—gaping shells indicate unhealthy specimens. The shells of lobster and shrimp should be hard. Fresh shellfish and crustacea don't have a strong, unpleasant smell.

SHOPPING FOR FRESH PRODUCE

> **Golden Rule:** Remember that even fresh produce can be contaminated with food poisoning germs. Always wrap loose produce in a bag in order to prevent contamination from getting on other foods in your grocery basket or cart.

Fresh produce isn't usually considered high-risk food, and at first, it's difficult to believe that foods such as fruits and salads can be a cause of food poisoning. However, since 1993, in the United States alone, there have been large outbreaks of salmonellosis linked to cantaloupes and alfalfa sprouts, *E. coli* O157 outbreaks associated with unpasteurized apple juice, extreme diarrhea illness caused by eating raspberries contaminated with *Cyclospora,* and a hepatitis A outbreak from contaminated strawberries. An outbreak of dysentery in Europe was linked to contaminated iceberg lettuce, and bean sprouts were implicated in a huge *E. coli* O157 outbreak in Japan.

How can produce become contaminated with animal germs? The explanations are very simple. The dirt in which the produce is grown may be treated with animal manures containing germs, or the crops may be irrigated with sewage-polluted water, or the harvested fruits and vegetables may even be washed in polluted water. Sometimes, crops such as apples fall from the tree onto ground where animals have been grazing. The outcome of any of these situations is that animal germs can be carried on the outer surface of any fresh produce. Also, fruit and vegetables, just like all other foods, may be contaminated by farm workers and food handlers who have enteric infections and who don't wash their hands properly. Oftentimes, in the United States as well as in other countries, toilets and sanitary facilities are not even available to workers out in the fields.

Prepackaged salads have also been found to sometimes contain the *Listeria* germ, although to date, these foods have not been associated with any known outbreaks of the illness listeriosis. In this instance, the contamination probably results from poor sanitation at the packaging factory.

SHOPPING FROM DELIS, SALAD BARS, AND BAKERIES

Delis and High-Risk Foods

Although most foods at a deli counter are precooked or ready to eat, much of what you buy here is classed as high-risk because it will not be cooked again and because it is often the type of food in which germs flourish.

Germs can easily grow in high-risk foods such as cold cooked meats and ready-to-eat potato salads and pasta salads. The germs may come from the food handlers or from the shoppers or from contact with contaminated raw foods. So food at a deli counter should be displayed in a refrigerated cabinet (at less than 40°F or 5°C), protected from customers by a glass screen, and completely separated from any raw foods that could contaminate the cooked foods.

> **Golden Rule:** Take extra care with high-risk foods.

Deli clerks should avoid handling the deli foods directly and should wear disposable gloves and use individual serving spoons for each food. All the ready-to-eat dishes should be replaced daily, but no sell-by dates are displayed here and consequently the same dishes may get put out day after day. If in doubt, ask the clerk when the dish was prepared.

Spit-roast chicken

Many deli counters offer freshly cooked spit-roast chicken for sale. Once the chicken is taken off the spit, it should be either eaten or refrigerated within two hours. Insist that you get a chicken directly off the spit—not one that has been sitting in a bag or a carton in the heated display counter for some time. Some stores label the cooked chicken with a two-hour time stamp so that you can see how long the chicken has been off the spit. Check out the spit-roasting procedure, too—if raw chickens are put on a spit above the already cooked chickens, the raw juices will drip onto the cooked chickens below and contaminate them.

Salad Bars

Salad bars contain many of the high-risk foods found at a deli counter but have the added risk of a self-service system. Self-serve systems in stores (and restaurants) are vulnerable to misuse, and it is almost impossible for the store to maintain control over what happens here. If you like to use the salad bar in your local supermarket, at least be aware of the following points.

First, the food in the salad bar should be kept at a refrigerated temperature of 40°F (5°C) or lower. Any food that is piled high above the container will probably be at room-air temperature, and only the food within the walls of the container remain cold. Second, there should always be a plastic sneeze-guard or shield in a direct line between the customer's face and the food in order to help prevent customers contaminating the food by coughing and sneezing over it. Third, tongs or a long-handled serving spoon should be available for each item so that customers will not need to touch the food with their hands. And finally, watch out for kids (and some adults) who are tempted to pick up foods with their fingers.

Bakeries

Breads, cookies, cakes, pastries, and pies are generally considered low-risk foods because the high temperatures at which they are baked destroys all germs. If problems do occur with baked goods, it is usually because something went wrong after the baking process. Often the fault lies with the food handlers—that is, the germs come from the hands of employees. Sometimes, problems occur because raw egg was used as a glaze and was not cooked long enough to kill *Salmonella* germs, or because meat fillings were not cooked thoroughly. Icings and cream fillings that are uncooked and meringues that are only partially cooked also pose problems.

Watch Out for Meringue

Meringue is made with a mixture of whipped egg white and sugar and baked at a low temperature for varying lengths of time, depending on whether it is a soft or hard meringue. Either way, the cooking process cannot be relied upon to kill the *Salmonella* germs that can be found inside eggs. The risk of food poisoning from *Salmonella* in meringues can be eliminated by using commercially prepared and pasteurized egg white (available in the frozen food or chilled food section of a supermarket). Using eggs from "*Salmonella*-free" chickens would also reduce the risk. Ask the bakery clerk about any baked goods with meringue.

The most important thing to watch out for at bakery counters is the way in which the bakery clerks handle the food. Again, plastic gloves and tongs should be used.

Self-service bread bins

Popular features in many stores are self-service bins containing items such as unwrapped bread rolls, bagels, and cookies. Just as at the salad bar, self-service can be a problem here, too, because customers are able to handle unwrapped foods and may contaminate the remaining foods by touching them with their hands or by coughing and sneezing over them. To lessen the risk of contamination, bins should be high enough off the floor so that people cannot bend over them, and each bin should have its own tongs, which can only be inserted into the bin through a hole just large enough for the baked item to pass through. This prevents customers from handling the breads and then putting them back in the bin. Trays of pastries are often displayed in glass cabinets. Here again, there is the potential for customers to handle unwrapped foods and cause contamination. Long-handled tongs should be used to select items and thus lessen the risk.

SHOPPING FOR REFRIGERATED AND FROZEN FOODS

Refrigerated Foods

Refrigerated cabinets and display cases contain a huge variety of packaged processed foods ranging from milk and orange juice to eggs, butter, yogurt, and cheese, to sliced meats and hot dogs, to smoked salmon, tofu, tortillas, and much more. All of these foods should be kept at refrigerated temperatures (less than 40°F or 5°C) and the cabinets and cases should be kept clean and neatly stacked. Don't purchase any items with damaged or leaky packaging, but do bring such items to the attention of store employees or the manager.

Golden Rule: Check the date stamp on all refrigerated and frozen foods.

Date stamps

On the outer packaging of all of these foods, you will see either a "sell-by" date, a "best if used by" date, or a "use-by" date. Here is what they mean:

- *"Sell-by" dates* tell the store how long to display this product. The food should still be safe well after this date. Deciding whether or not to eat foods beyond their sell-by dates is a matter of judgment. High-risk foods should be consumed within two or three days of a sell-by date. Check out page 78 for how long to keep these products at home.
- *"Best if used by"* or *"Best before"* dates refer to the flavor and quality of the product, *not* to its safety. So while you may safely eat a product a few days past this date, its taste might not be so good.
- *"Use-by" dates* should be taken seriously. This date reflects the manufacturer's advice on when the food will lose its quality. Do not eat foods beyond this date.

It is illegal for stores to sell any items beyond their sell-by or use-by dates. These stamps should be the consumer's ally in shopping for safe food, but they are confusing. *Only the use-by date offers clear information on food safety.* If the food industry would adopt a universal standard, such as an "eat-by" date, the message would be clear to both consumers and retailers.

How shelves are stacked

Stores stack refrigerated foods on the shelves from front to back with the older stock (close to the date limit) at the front and the most recently received stock (with a longer date limit) at the back. If you shop infrequently or do a big shop to last you a week or more, then select items with the longest date limit from the back of the shelf. This way you get a longer period to keep these products safely at home.

Milk

Almost all the milk sold in stores is pasteurized, meaning that it has been heated to a very high temperature for a few seconds. This destroys most of the germs without altering the flavor of the milk, and any germs that survive are reduced to very low levels so that the milk is safe. But milk can be on the store shelves for up to two weeks, and there have been reports that some milk may have unacceptably high levels of germs by that time. This means that the milk quickly goes "off" once you've got it home. To avoid this, buy the milk with the longest date limit stacked at the back of the shelf.

Eggs

Always open egg cartons to check the eggs, and reject any carton containing cracked or dirty eggs. Eggs sold in the United States should be less than two weeks old and must show a use-by date.

Fruit juices

Because contaminated, unpasteurized apple juice has been linked with outbreaks of *E. coli* O157 illness, it is safer to buy pasteurized apple cider and other juices. Juices prepared at home from carefully washed fruit or vegetables should be consumed immediately. For additional safety, heat unpasteurized juices to the boiling point for a few seconds.

Frozen Foods

Freezers should be maintained at a temperature of 0°F (−18°C) or lower and should be clean and neatly stacked. Watch for date stamps and any signs that foods may have thawed and then refrozen.

Signs of thawing and refreezing

Thawing and refreezing are major dangers for frozen foods because bacteria germs can multiply during the thaw and survive the refreezing. The food then becomes contaminated with a lot of germs and can cause problems, especially if the food is an item that doesn't need cooking. Telltale signs include large ice crystals, solid areas of ice, discolored or dried-out food, and misshapen cartons or packages. Reject any doubtful items, and tell the management that there are some problems in the freezer.

SHOPPING FOR CANNED, DRIED, AND BOTTLED FOODS

These foods are classed as low-risk foods. As long as these foods are stored correctly, germs can't thrive in them because they are either too dry, too acidic, or too sugary, or they contain preservatives or have been baked or subjected to a high-temperature canning or bottling process. In other words, these foods have gone through a commercial preservation process, much like the ones described in Chapter 13. Even so, all these foods require careful storage and have a recommended use-by date.

Many jars now have a tamper-proof seal, and the item should be rejected if the seal is broken. Some jars, such as those containing baby food, have a button in the lid that indicates whether the seal is good.

> *Golden Rule:* Check for dented cans and damaged seals and packaging. Never purchase any item if you think the packaging may have been tampered with in any way.

Canned Foods and Drinks

Don't buy or use food from any cans with swollen sides or ends, damaged seals or seams, rust, dents, leaks, or foamy or bad-smelling contents. In the past, failures in commercial canning procedures have resulted in outbreaks of botulism, but today botulism is more often associated with home-canning practices. (Information on home canning is given in Chapter 13.)

The toxin produced by *Clostridium botulinum,* the bacteria that causes botulism, is lethal, and swallowing as little as 0.1 gram of contaminated food can cause illness. In the United States, most outbreaks of botulism in adults are caused not by eating store-bought foods, but by eating home-canned or fermented vegetables. In Alaska and Canada, however, home-canned fish products most often cause botulism. The most common form of botulism in the United States today is infant botulism in babies under a year old, and it is often caused by honey and corn syrup contaminated with naturally occurring spores. The infant immature immune system may not be able to prevent spore germination inside the intestinal tract and the resulting illness. Honey and corn syrup are not a source of the preformed toxin.

Dried Foods and Drinks

When selecting dried packaged foods such as cereals and other grain products, sugar, flour, and rice, and dried fruits and vegetables, make sure that the packaging is dry and undamaged. Dampness or mold is a sign that the food is spoiling and should not be eaten. Holes or tears in the packaging may be signs of damage caused by insects or rodents.

Bottled Foods and Drinks

Bottled foods and drinks are highly preserved and should remain safe as long as they are unopened. Reject any items that show signs of cloudiness at the bottom of the container; mold growth, which can look like fluffy balls floating or carpeting the surface; an unexpected "yeasty" smell; or bubbles rising slowly from the bottom of the bottle. The bubbles and the yeasty smell are signs that the food is spoiling because germs have caused the food to begin fermenting.

Food Abuse

The deliberate sabotage of foods is a relatively new and particularly nasty crime. Medicines, supermarket foods, and even foods served at social functions in settings such as universities have all been the subject of criminal abuse.

8

THE CHECK-OUT AND GETTING THE FOOD HOME SAFELY

> **Golden Rule:** Minimize the time from store to home storage.

At last—you've finished your shopping. Now all you have to do is check out, get your groceries bagged, pay the bill, and you're out of there. Right?

Unfortunately, at the very last, foods may be contaminated by contact with a dirty counter at the check-out and at the hands of the check-out staff. The staff themselves are also at risk from contact with raw foods. They, too, get meat juices on their hands when a leaky package comes by. The check-out area should be kept very clean with an antibacterial cleaner, and there should be antibacterial handiwipes available here, both for the staff and for the customers.

If it's summertime and the temperature outside and in your car is soaring, you should take a few extra minutes to think about how to get all those refrigerated and frozen items home without them undergoing a potentially dangerous warming on the way. The best solution is to take your cooler or cool bags and ice packs with you to the store and have all the frozen, refrigerated, and high-risk items put straight into the cooler at the check-out. Alternatively, place these items into your cooler as soon as you get your groceries to your car. There are also some insulated plastic grocery bags designed especially to keep foods cool. At the very least, have the bagger put all the cool and cold items together in double paper or plastic bags, both for some insulation protection and so that you can put a high priority on getting these bags unpacked and into your refrigerator or freezer as soon as you get home.

Having taken so much care in the selection and bagging of your food, it is important to transport it home as quickly as possible, especially in the summertime. On hot days, the trunk of the car can reach temperatures in the danger zone for many foods, and the temperature of the food itself will quickly begin to climb if left in these conditions. Using a cooler will allow you more time to get the food home safely.

It is often not until you get home and unpack your shopping that you are able to make a close inspection of your purchases. At this point, you may become aware that something looks or smells bad. If this happens, either return the purchase to the store immediately or phone them and tell them what you've found. The important thing is that if you have any concerns, pay attention to your instincts and don't eat the food or even taste it. Remember the safe-food mantra: *If in doubt, throw it out.*

PART FOUR

HOW TO PREVENT FOOD POISONING IN YOUR KITCHEN

9

STORING FOOD AT HOME

The first step in preventing food poisoning at home is to learn how to store foods properly in order to ensure that they remain in good condition until you're ready to eat them.

REFRIGERATED AND FROZEN FOODS

As soon as you bring groceries home, your first priority should be to get frozen and chilled foods back into a freezer or a refrigerator as quickly as possible because once these foods begin to thaw and warm, any germs that are present can multiply rapidly. These germs will not all be killed by any subsequent chilling or freezing.

> *Golden Rule:* Frozen foods that have thawed should never be refrozen until after thorough cooking. Foods such as ice cream and other frozen desserts should not be refrozen if they accidentally thaw.

Using Your Refrigerator Wisely

Refrigerators should be run at 40°F (5°C) or lower, and the only way to be sure about the temperature is to use a refrigerator thermometer. Very few domestic refrigerators have a built-in thermometer, and the dial for adjusting the temperature to "cooler" or "less cool" does not usually have a temperature gauge. The temperature inside a refrigerator can rapidly rise to almost room temperature under certain circumstances—for example, if you leave the door open on a hot day while you load the refrigerator. Once you close the door, it may take many hours for the temperature to cool down again.

In general, the coldest area in the refrigerator is at the back, and the warmest area is by the door. Keep a refrigerator thermometer near the front, and check that the temperature stays between 35° and 40°F (2°–5°C). Refrigerator thermometers and combined freezer/refrigerator thermometers are quite inexpensive and can be obtained from some kitchen stores and from restaurant supply stores.

Do not line refrigerator shelves, as this cuts down on air circulation and stops proper cooling. Store cooked and ready-to-eat foods above raw meat and fish so that there is no chance that the raw foods can drip contaminated juices onto the cooked foods. Place raw meat, poultry, or fish on a plate or a dish and loosely cover with plastic wrap. Store eggs in the main body of the refrigerator where temperatures are coldest, not in the door. Salad greens, green vegetables, and fruit can be kept in the storage compartments at the bottom of the refrigerator. Newer models offer a choice between low-humidity storage for hard fruits and root vegetables and high-humidity storage for salad items. Foods containing low levels of preservative, such as jams, jellies, and mayonnaise, require refrigeration after they have been opened. Read the storage instructions on the label carefully.

Dairy foods

All dairy foods should be stored in the refrigerator. Butter, cheese, whipped cream, and yogurt can also be frozen. In the refrigerator, milk can be stored for one week, half-and-half and cream for four days, hard cheese for three to four weeks and soft cheese for one week, sour cream and yogurt for two weeks.

Baby foods

Don't fool around with baby foods. Babies are a high-risk group for food poisoning, and they can get very sick. Strictly follow the use-by date on jars, cans, and formula for babies. Once opened, jars and cans of food should be refrigerated and used within one to two days. Formula can be made up and refrigerated but must be used within twenty-four hours.

Using Your Freezer Wisely

Domestic freezers operate at 0°F (−18°C). Foods placed in the freezer should be already frozen or at least chilled. Putting warm foods into the freezer can cause other frozen foods to warm up and thaw a little. Thawing and refreezing damages the food quality and gives food poisoning germs a chance to multiply in the food while it is partially thawed. Place foods such as breads in freezer bags to prevent drying and freezer damage, and use a marker pen to label and date foods. Some foods suffer damage to texture and flavor (commonly known as freezer burn) if they are kept frozen for too long. These foods include hamburger, mackerel, salmon, turkey, pork, creamed foods, sauces, custards, gravies, and puddings. Check storage instructions for all foods that you plan to freeze.

Power outages

Short breaks in the electricity supply won't affect the food in the freezer, but if the power cut lasts more than a few hours, it's a good idea to pack any spaces in the freezer with newspaper and towels and then keep the door shut, in order to slow the thawing process. Power cuts of twelve hours or more will usually result in a thaw and the loss of much of the frozen food. Do not refreeze any completely thawed items until after you cook them first.

Storage Guidelines for Refrigerated and Frozen Foods

Food	Refrigerator	Freezer
Fresh eggs	3–4 weeks	No
Egg white/yolk	4 days	4 months
Commercial mayonnaise	Refrigerate after opening	No
Frozen dinners	No	4 months
Hamburger and other ground meats	1–2 days	3–4 months
Vacuum-packed meats	2 weeks if unopened. Once opened, eat within 2–3 days.	2 months
Hot dogs and cold meats	2 weeks in sealed vacuum pack. Once opened, eat within 4 days.	3–4 months
Fresh meat	3 days	4–6 months
Fresh poultry	1–2 days	9 months
Fresh fish and shellfish	2 days	2–3 months

Safe Thawing

There are three ways to safely thaw frozen food at home:

1. *In a refrigerator:* Put the frozen item on a tray or dish on the bottom shelf to prevent the juices from dripping or splashing on other foods. Allow a day or more to thaw large items such as turkeys and roasts.
2. *As part of the cooking process:* Use this method only for small items such as vegetables, shrimps, and pie shells. Allow a longer cooking time for frozen items. Not safe for big items, and not recommended for hamburger patties, which may not cook thoroughly.

3. *In a microwave:* Only food that is going to be cooked immediately should be thawed in the microwave. Not safe for big items.

Golden Rule: Make it the law—use the fridge to thaw.

CANNED, BOTTLED, AND DRIED FOODS

Canned, bottled, and dried food and drink can be safely stored for long periods at room temperature and away from sunlight, but it is still important to regularly check the expiration dates. Some canned and bottled foods need to be refrigerated once opened, so look for storage information on the label. Once opened, foods should not be left in unlined cans, because oxidation of the metal can cause the food to go bad. It's better to store leftovers from opened cans in clean, covered storage containers.

Keep dried fruits and vegetables, cereals, pastas, and other grain products, sugar, flour, rice, cookies, and snack foods in their own packaging, or transfer them to clean, dry, airtight containers. Also keep these foods dry, because any moisture in the food or on the packaging and even prolonged high humidity may cause these foods to spoil. Typically, mold or mildew are signs that these foods have gotten damp and have spoiled.

FRUITS AND VEGETABLES

Fresh fruits and vegetables have a limited shelf life, but proper storage will help to keep them in good condition. Avoid warm, moist storage conditions and condensation, both of which will encourage bacteria and mold to grow and cause spoilage. Open plastic wraps to allow air circulation. Most fruits and vegetables can be stored in the refrigerator, although tropical fruits such as bananas and pineapples are best stored in a cool place (50°F or 10°C) but not at refrigerator temperatures. Store potatoes in a cool, dry place and away from light.

BREADS AND PASTRIES

Fresh bread, pastries, and confectioneries have a very short shelf life before they become stale and moldy. Any items containing fresh or synthetic cream, custard, egg custard, or any meat products should be refrigerated and consumed within two to three days. All other breads, cakes, and cookies should be stored in a cool, dry place. Condensation or moisture inside the plastic wrapping causes bread to go moldy very quickly.

DECIDING WHEN TO REJECT FOOD

Golden Rule: If in doubt, throw it out.

Sometimes you have to decide whether a food item is still safe to eat. Foods can become spoiled for a number of reasons, such as damage to the packaging, poor storage conditions, and age. Signs of spoiled foods are easy to spot: discoloration, the presence of mold (both the slimy and the hairy varieties), bad or "off" odors, and fermentation (gas bubbles and a yeasty smell). Reject and discard any foods that show either signs of spoilage or damaged containers, especially canned and bottled foods, where damage and spoilage may indicate the presence of the bacteria that causes botulism. There is more information on how to dispose of suspect cans in Chapter 13.

Mold

Many people often simply remove the layer of mold from cheese or jam and continue to eat the remaining food. This is not a safe practice, because invisible toxins from the mold can spread into the food beyond the area of the visible mold. So even when you eat a portion of the food that isn't moldy, you may still be getting a dose of the toxin. This leads to questions about the safety of food-processing techniques that utilize molds for their flavor, such as the production of blue cheeses. These techniques use molds in a controlled way to minimize toxin production, and of course, such foods are usually only consumed in very small quantities.

Molds, Toxins, and Cancer

When molds grow on or in foods, they can produce myco-toxins in the food, some of which may cause bad allergy reactions and possibly even some types of cancer. Moldy feeds cause cancer and birth deformities in farm animals.

Food Poisoning Germs

Unfortunately, food that contains food poisoning germs does not show any signs of their presence. There is not necessarily any relationship between signs of food spoilage and the presence of food poisoning germs. In other words, don't believe that food is free from germs that cause food poisoning just because it doesn't show any signs of spoilage, such as a bad smell. Food that is contaminated with huge numbers of *Salmonella* or *E. coli* can look and smell perfectly normal. If in any doubt, the safest action is just to discard the food— and do not be tempted "to taste it to make sure."

10

PREPARING AND COOKING FOOD SAFELY

> **Golden Rule:** Guard against cross-contamination.

Safe food handling, preparation, and cooking are critical to reducing the risk of causing or acquiring food poisoning. With the knowledge that so many raw foods coming into the kitchen can be contaminated with food poisoning germs, it is essential to prevent those germs from getting onto other foods or onto your hands and directly to your mouth.

RAW FOODS OF ANIMAL ORIGIN

Greatest care should be taken with raw foods of animal origin—all meat, poultry, eggs, and fish. The safest way to deal with these foods is to assume that they *are* contaminated with food poisoning germs and to always take the following precautions.

First, before starting to handle any foods, wash your hands thoroughly (see Chapter 14). Also, wash your hands again after handling raw foods and between handling raw foods and other foods. Second, wear a clean apron: It protects your clothes, and it protects the food from any germs on your clothing. Third, do not smoke, drink, or eat while preparing food, especially raw food, because you run the risk of carrying food poisoning germs on your fingers directly to your mouth, and you might also contaminate the food with germs from your mouth and face via your fingers. Finally, refrigerate prepared foods, especially those of animal origins, including egg batters, if there is a delay between preparation and cooking. Also refrigerate foods while they are being marinated.

PREVENTING CROSS-CONTAMINATION

Do not allow raw foods, especially meat and fish, to touch other foods such as salads or fruits, which are not going to be cooked. Even the juices from raw meat and fish can carry food poisoning germs and contaminate other foods. This process of germs being carried from raw foods to other foods is called cross-contamination. And it can happen when food poisoning germs get onto your hands or onto cutting boards, countertops, sponges, dishcloths, scrubbers, and brushes. That's why it's important to keep all kitchen work surfaces, utensils, and cooking equipment hygienically clean. All kitchen items that have been in contact with raw foods should be washed in hot soapy water or in the dishwasher, and all kitchen surfaces should be cleaned and sanitized. (More information on keeping the kitchen hygienically clean is given in Chapter 14.)

To minimize the risk of cross-contamination, keep the preparation of raw foods separate from that of other food. If possible, complete the preparation of raw foods, and then remove all items that have been in contact with the raw foods, clean and sanitize the counters, and wash your hands before starting on the preparation of other foods. Also, keep a cutting board for raw meat and another for vegetables and fruits. (For more information about cutting boards, see Chapter 14.)

If you need to rinse a cut of meat, poultry, or fish, do this carefully in a bowl of cold water placed in the sink. Pour away the rinse water carefully to avoid splashing the surrounding areas.

Wash the bowl in hot soapy water and sanitize the sink area. Rinsing under a running tap is not recommended, as it causes splashing and contamination of the sink and surrounding area with germs.

EGGS

There is a lot of new advice about preparing and eating eggs, because *Salmonella* bacteria have been found both in egg yolk and in egg white. When preparing eggs, and especially when beating or whisking them, try to avoid splashing the yolks or the whites, as they can cause cross-contamination and carry the *Salmonella* to other surfaces or other foods. Clean and sanitize any raw egg splashes. Don't taste uncooked foods such as cake and cookie batters that contain raw egg, and don't pass the bowl over to the kids to lick the raw batter. It's a good idea to use pasteurized eggs for recipes in which the eggs will not be cooked thoroughly—for example, meringues, mousses, Caesar salad dressing, hollandaise and béarnaise sauces, egg nog, and mayonnaise.

COOKING FOOD TO MAKE IT SAFE

Golden Rule: Cook food thoroughly to make it safe.

Cooking food to the right internal temperature is the strongest weapon in the fight against food poisoning germs. Cooking destroys most food poisoning germs and makes the food safe to eat, so long as it is served quickly or rapidly cooled and refrigerated. You need to take care with each of the different cooking methods used in the home in order to ensure that food really is cooked thoroughly.

Internal Cooking Temperatures

The only way to know whether food has reached the right internal temperature is to check it with a thermometer. If you don't have a thermometer, cook all meats until the juices run clear, not pink, and the meat is not raw when you cut into it.

Instant-read thermometers

Instant-read thermometers are the most accurate and can be used to check the temperature of anything that is cooked, either in the oven or microwave or on the stove top or grill. And because this type of thermometer is calibrated to record temperatures in a range from zero to 220°F (−18° to 104°C), it can also be used to check the temperatures of cold food.

Unlike the less accurate "meat thermometers" that are left in a roast as it cooks, the instant-read thermometer should be plunged into the thickest part of the food until it hits the pan or the bone, and then withdrawn slightly. After about fifteen seconds, the dial should register an accurate reading. After reading, the thermometer must be removed from the food or it will be destroyed by the heat. After use, the thermometer stem should always be sanitized to prevent transferring germs from one food to another via the thermometer. The easiest way to sanitize these thermometers is to use an alcohol wipe (available from a pharmacy), but you can also use a dilute bleach solution. They should not be immersed in water or put in the dishwasher. Kitchen stores sell basic instant-read thermometers for about $12, and electronic models for about $28. Restaurant supply stores offer lower prices.

The 160°F (70°C) temperature

In the past, a confusing number of different internal temperatures have been offered for different foods, and it was difficult to remember just what temperature to use. In fact, there is only one important temperature to remember—160°F (70°C). This is the lowest temperature that reliably kills food poisoning germs and destroys heat-sensitive toxins. All meat and poultry, stuffings containing meat products, leftovers, and stuffed meats and pastas should be cooked to this minimum internal temperature.

Toxins

Some germs, such as *Staphylococcus,* produce toxins in food that are not always destroyed by heat. In this case, cooking cannot be relied on to make the food safe. The need to keep food safe at *all* stages of storage, preparation, and cooking is critical.

Partial or interrupted cooking

Some recipes call for the partial cooking of a food with completion of the cooking process at a later time. If the partial cooking does not reach the critical temperature of 160°F or above, bacteria may be able to multiply quickly in the warm food. If the subsequent cooking is not thorough, this leaves the food heavily contaminated. It is safer for all cooking to be completed in a single operation.

Slow cookers

It is important to ensure that any slow cooker or Crock-Pot reaches and maintains a food temperature above the minimum 160°F. Check this by using an instant-read thermometer.

SAFETY TIPS FOR COOKING

Cook fish until the flesh flakes with a fork. Cook eggs and egg dishes until the yolks and whites are firm, never runny. Cook stuffings separately from meat and poultry, and then stuff the food once both the meat and the stuffing are cooked. This is because stuffing meat and poultry before cooking can insulate the internal surfaces and prevent thorough cooking. Batters and breadings can also insulate the food they cover and can prevent complete cooking, so take care to ensure that these items are thoroughly cooked, too. And dispose of any leftover batter—don't be tempted to save it for another meal—it might grow too many germs in the meantime.

Tips for Cooking Mollusks

Mollusks are a group of shellfish that includes mussels, scallops, clams, oysters, and cockles. Before cooking, the shells should be tightly closed, or if open, they should close quickly when tapped. Discard any shells that are cracked or open and stay open when tapped—these are signs of a sick or dead mollusk. Wash the shellfish thoroughly in running water. In order to ensure that any fecal virus contaminants are killed, especially hepatitis A virus, cook mollusks to an internal temperature of 194°F (90°C)— roughly equivalent to steaming for four minutes. Do not serve any shells that remain closed after cooking.

Oysters

Many oyster beds around the world are known to be contaminated with germs from human sewage pollution, and as a result, raw oysters can no longer be considered a safe delicacy. Some of the oyster beds along the coast of the southern United States are even contaminated with the cholera germ, thought to have been transported to the region in the bilge waters of visiting ships.

TASTING THE SAFE WAY

Many people like to check on the taste of a dish during cooking or preparation. TV chefs are always seen tasting their dishes—and often the wrong way, by dipping a finger or using the same spoon several times. The safe way to taste food is to use a clean spoon and never put the same spoon back into the food without washing it first. Dipping a finger into the food or using a spoon several times can cause direct contamination of the food with germs from the skin or mouth.

MAKING RECIPES SAFE

The purpose of this chapter is to offer guidelines on cooking safe food in your kitchen and reducing the risk of food poisoning. Consequently, some of the information given here differs from recipe instructions found in cookbooks, magazines, and recipe cards. The fact that some dishes undoubtedly carry a risk of illness is almost never mentioned in recipe books. As a result, many recipes still list raw uncooked egg as an ingredient in dishes such as homemade mousses and mayonnaise.

You'll find that many recipes can be safely modified, for example, by substituting pasteurized egg for raw or undercooked egg and by adjusting the cooking temperatures to the minimum temperatures recommended in this chapter. If the recipe cannot be safely modified, then you need to decide whether this is a good recipe for you to use.

Of course, it's up to you whether you want to take the risk of eating raw egg and other raw or undercooked foods of animal origin. That decision should be based on factors such as the current state of health and the age of yourself, your loved ones, and other guests at your table. But remember, "good food" must also be "safe food."

COOKING ON THE GRILL

Cooking outdoors on the grill or barbecue is a very popular summertime activity and is often the center of a social event for families and friends. But many cases of food poisoning have been traced to food hygiene errors in the grilling procedures. Perhaps the very fact that barbecuing is a outdoor social event leads people to forget that the same hygiene rules apply to this type of cooking activity as to all others. One of the major problems with grilling is that food is often overcooked on the outside but undercooked on the inside. Undercooked grilled meat, especially chicken and hamburgers, is a food poisoning hazard that is especially dangerous to children and other high-risk groups.

Safety Tips for Grilling and Barbecuing

- Marinate all food items in the refrigerator.
- Keep foods in the refrigerator until it is time to grill them.
- Cook foods thoroughly—cut into pieces of meat or fish to check that they are cooked through and are not pink. Better still, use an instant-read thermometer to check on the internal temperature.
- Thaw frozen foods before grilling, especially items such as beef patties.
- Use clean utensils.
- Put cooked items onto a *clean* serving dish. Do not put them back onto a dish that held raw foods.
- Do not use leftover marinade from the raw foods to flavor the cooked foods.
- Teach your kids to ask for well-cooked hamburgers and to reject any that look pink inside.

MICROWAVE COOKING

Microwave ovens are found in most home kitchens in the United States. Cooks like microwaving because it is clean, quick, and convenient. In addition to keeping the internal surfaces of the microwave clean and sanitized, here are a few points to be aware of in order to ensure that microwaved food is safe from food poisoning germs.

How Microwaves Cook Food

In microwave cooking, heat is generated in the food by the microwaves vibrating the food molecules, causing friction and heat. The food cooks itself and continues cooking even when the power is off. Like conventional ovens, microwaves have hot and cold spots that may cause uneven heating, and if there is no built-in turntable, you'll need to turn or stir the food to ensure that all of it is heated throughout to a high enough temperature to kill food poisoning germs.

Power levels and wattage

Microwaves work on varying power levels, depending on the wattage of the oven. The different power settings on most microwaves—high (100 percent), medium (50 percent), defrost (30 percent), and low (10 percent)—indicate the amount of energy produced in bursts in a given time. In other words, high means that power is being produced during 100 percent of the cooking time; medium, about 50 percent of the time; defrost, about 30 percent of the time; and low, 10 percent of the time. Different models have different settings, so be sure to check your user's manual.

Cooking Tips

For microwave cooking, you need to add a minimum of 25 degrees Fahrenheit (or 14 degrees centigrade) to conventional internal cooking temperatures to ensure that food is cooked safely. So, the microwave minimum internal temperature is 185°F (85°C) instead of the 160°F (70°C) for conventional cooking. For roasting meat or poultry in the microwave, use an instant-read thermometer (see page 85). *Never* use a conventional metal meat thermometer. Some combination ovens have a built-in temperature probe. If the microwave doesn't have a turntable, rotate or stir the food midway through cooking to help spread the heat evenly throughout. Cooked foods should be allowed to stand for two minutes after cooking so that all parts of the food heat to the recommended internal temperature. For refrigerated entrees in sealed packaging, always follow instructions and timings on the package to ensure that the food gets to the required internal temperature. For reheating home-cooked foods, also make sure that the minimum internal temperature is reached.

Thawing Tips

Defrost power is about 30 percent output, but certain thinly sliced meats and fish may need low (10 percent) power so that the edges do not start cooking before the insides are fully thawed. Small chickens and cuts of meat thaw easily, but first place them on sheets of paper towels to absorb the juices. Check inside poultry to see that it is free from ice before cooking. Because the food may have started to warm up during thawing, it should be cooked as soon as it has defrosted.

Materials and Packaging

Almost any heatproof dish or plate can be used in the microwave as long as it's not metal and has no metallic rim or pattern. Glass, china, glazed earthenware, paper, and rigid plastics that do not melt at low temperatures can be used. Check the user's manual for advice on microwave utensils. Microwave plastic wrap can be used to cover dishes and bowls, but food experts recommend that the wrap not be in contact with hot foods of a high fat content. This is because of concern about chemicals leaching out of the plastic and into the food. Pierce a few holes in the plastic wrap or turn back a small piece to let out steam. Wax paper can also be used to cover and safely touch foods.

11

SERVING FOOD SAFELY AND DEALING WITH LEFTOVERS

Even when food has been thoroughly cooked, it is still very important that it be handled and served safely to prevent it from becoming contaminated with germs again. Contamination might come from contact with other raw foods, dirty utensils and preparation surfaces, unwashed hands, coughs and sneezes, household pets, or pests such as flies. As a general rule, it is best to handle food as little as possible once it has been cooked. The time between preparation and consumption is crucial because hygiene failures that occur at this stage will not be corrected by any further cooking.

Once food is ready to serve, avoid cross-contamination by using only clean serving dishes and utensils and by washing your hands immediately before serving the food. Even though your hands are clean, try not to touch the food. Use serving utensils wherever possible, and invite others who are helping themselves to food to do the same. Also, make sure that the food is protected from pets and pests.

The Two-Hour Rule

Never allow cooked and prepared foods to stand unrefrigerated for more than two hours before the food is either

---

93

eaten, cooked, recooked, or cooled and refrigerated. Food poisoning germs can multiply quickly in food left out of the refrigerator at temperatures between 40°F and 140°F (5°–60°C). In hot summer temperatures, and even in over-heated houses in winter, the two-hour rule should be cut back to one hour maximum.

SERVING A SAFE BUFFET

Buffets can be a real challenge to serving safe food. Buffets often involve high-risk protein foods of animal origin or foods that take a lot of handling during preparation. The food sits around for several hours during service. Finally, when people help themselves to the food, there's always the added risk of contamination.

Hot food can be kept hot at the stove or by serving it from chafing dishes or warming trays. The food should be kept at an internal temperature of at least 140°F (60°C). Use an instant-read thermometer (see Chapter 10) to check on this. But don't keep food at this temperature for longer than two hours (remember the two-hour rule). After two hours, any leftover food should be thrown away if there is any doubt about temperature control during the buffet. It may seem wasteful to throw away apparently "good" food, but food that has been through a preparation-and-cooking process and then has been held at a temperature dipping below 140°F for two hours in a buffet (especially a self-serve buffet) may already be on the limits of safety for germ load. Any further storage will allow the germ levels to increase and make the food unsafe.

Cold food should be kept on ice and served cold. Replace the ice as it melts; otherwise, the food will start to warm up. Keep the food covered and protected as much as possible.

If you're planning a self-serve buffet, make sure that you provide enough clean serving utensils so that guests are not tempted to serve themselves with their own used eating utensils, thereby possibly contaminating the food with their own germs. And guard against double dipping (see page 102).

DEALING WITH LEFTOVERS

As mentioned earlier, all cooked foods should either be eaten immediately or be kept hot at 140°F or higher for no more than two hours, or they should be cooled and refrigerated within two hours of cooking. Thus, any germs that survived the cooking process or were accidentally introduced after cooking do not have time to multiply to unsafe levels.

However, it can be quite difficult to cool foods this rapidly without the kind of equipment available in commercial kitchens. Cooling techniques that may seem obvious but should be avoided include putting hot food directly into the refrigerator (causing everything else inside to heat up), leaving uncovered hot food to cool at an open window (making it vulnerable to contamination from sources such as pets and pests), and leaving hot food sitting in a pan on top of the stove or in the oven for hours (the food cools so slowly that any germs that survived the cooking process have time to recover and regrow).

Golden Rule: Don't get sick. Cool it quick.

Tips for Cooling Hot Food

The key to cooling food rapidly is to remember that the smaller the volume of food and the larger its surface area, the quicker it will cool. The aim is to reduce the food temperature to 40°F (5°C) or less (refrigerator temperatures). Check the temperature with an instant-read thermometer (Chapter 10). Soups and thick foods such as stew, chili, polenta, and pudding can be cooled by pouring them into large, clean, shallow containers sitting in ice. Stir the food as it cools so that no warm spots are left. Cut up large pieces of hot food into smaller pieces, and divide large pans of hot food into smaller, clean containers on ice. Once the food has cooled, loosely cover the containers and place them on a shelf in the refrigerator so that air can circulate around them for further cooling.

Reheating Cooked Food

People are often confused about whether reheating food is a safe practice. The safest practice is to reheat food only once and to ensure that it reaches a minimum internal temperature of 160°F (70°C) within a two-hour cooking period. Food reheated in a microwave should reach a temperature of 185°F (85°C) and be allowed to stand for two minutes after reheating so that the heat spreads evenly throughout the food. Any food that is not consumed after reheating once should be discarded.

> *Golden Rule:* Reheat leftovers only once, and make sure the internal temperature reaches 160°F.

Disposal of Unwanted Food

Food that's to be thrown out should be placed in the trash quickly so that no one eats it by mistake. Foods that are not fit for human consumption are usually not good for pets either; and if it makes the pets sick, they may pass the infection on to the humans around them. Infection can be transmitted through vomit, feces, or even by just stroking the animal. Germs that are excreted in pet feces can contaminate their fur and, in turn, be transferred to your hands as you stroke your pet. Seal the food in the trash, and use pestproof trash containers in order to avoid attracting flies and rats to the area. Empty the kitchen trash frequently so that pests will not be drawn to the kitchen.

12

COOKING FOR HOLIDAYS AND PARTIES

Golden Rule: Have a happy, healthy, safe-food holiday.

There is often an increase in food poisoning around holidays such as the Fourth of July, Thanksgiving, and Christmas. This is attributed in part to the increased consumption of meat and poultry at these times and to the problems associated with handling these foods safely. The preparation of big holiday meals can undoubtedly put a huge strain on the limited facilities of a domestic kitchen, forcing unintentional errors in safe-food practice and perhaps triggering an outbreak of food poisoning. And few things are more embarrassing than having a social event ruined by a food poisoning incident. The following guidelines will help you to safely prepare for a range of special food events.

Cater within Your Comfort Zone

In other words, try to tailor the number of people that you are catering for to what you feel you can comfortably cope with within the limitations of your kitchen. For example, will you be able to find refrigerator space for all the items that need to be kept cool? Keep in mind that anyone who is ill with any form of vomiting or diarrhea illness should not be preparing or serving food because of the risk of contaminating the food with their own germs. So, if you are unfortunate enough to get sick at this busy time, either arrange for someone else to take over all of the catering preparations or postpone or cancel the event rather than risk causing other people to become sick, too. Remember that some of the guests may be higher-risk individuals for food poisoning, and plan the menus with this in mind. More advice on cooking for higher-risk individuals is given in Chapters 15 and 16.

THE BIG HOLIDAY MEAL

Typically, the holiday meal involves the preparation of many different food items, including appetizers, vegetables and salads, and a number of different desserts, as well as a turkey, ham, or other large cut of meat. Preparing and handling the meat often leads to cross-contamination of germs onto hands and other surfaces in the kitchen and then onto other foods. So, there are a number of things you need to be alert to during the preparation of such a meal.

Start by helping yourself—get as much of the preparation done in advance as possible and freeze the items until required. Thaw frozen meat or poultry slowly in the refrigerator, and allow sufficient time for this. A large bird can take several days to defrost. A large roast or turkey usually takes four to seven hours per pound to thaw, and a small roast or bird takes three to five hours per pound. Put the frozen meat or poultry on a dish or tray on the bottom shelf of the refrigerator to prevent the thawed juices from dripping or spilling. Remove any plastic wrapping, but keep the frozen item loosely covered and make sure it isn't touching other foods. Once thawed, remove giblets from the turkey, keep it refrigerated, and cook it within twenty-four hours. Wipe up any spillage of raw meat juices in the refrigerator or on kitchen surfaces using dilute bleach or an antibacterial kitchen cleaner.

Do not refreeze partially defrosted raw foods of animal origin without cooking them first. And always wash your hands thoroughly after handling raw meat or poultry. Rinse all fruit and vegetables under a running tap. Try to avoid dishes that use uncooked raw egg; substitute pasteurized egg instead.

Calculating the turkey cooking time

Calculate the cooking time by using the bird's weight. The guide is roughly twenty minutes per pound plus an extra twenty minutes at 325°F (160°C), although the cooking time per pound decreases with very heavy birds. Cook to a *minimum* internal temperature of 160°F. Cook any stuffing separately from the bird, and add it before serving. If you cook a roast but are not planning to eat it right away, remove it from the oven, cool it quickly, and refrigerate (advice on cooling is given in Chapter 11).

PARTIES AT HOME

Whether you're serving a sit-down meal, a buffet, or just trays of finger foods, plan the meal carefully in advance and consider whether you will need the use of extra refrigerator or freezer space. Neighbors can often help out with extra space on these occasions. Keep the recipes and menus simple. It is far better to serve good, simple food that has been safely prepared than a fancy menu that stretches your abilities to keep the food safe.

Start by asking your butcher or meat clerk to do as much of the raw meat preparation as possible. This way you can avoid having to debone, trim, or cut up the meat or poultry in your own kitchen, and you limit the risk of cross-contamination. And of course, always buy the food from a reputable supplier. Do as much of the preparation as possible in advance, and freeze any prepared foods. This relieves the pressure of getting everything done at the last minute and also reduces the risk of cross-contamination. Keep the kitchen tidy, and keep raw foods separate from all other foods.

Advanced preparation of foods that will not be frozen should take place within twelve to twenty four hours of the party, and all the items should be refrigerated. Avoid recipes containing raw or undercooked foods of animal origin, and substitute raw egg with pasteurized egg. Carefully wash all fruits, vegetables, and salad greens under a running tap, and use only clean drinking water for ice cubes and drinks and for all food preparation. Hot food should always be served quickly after cooking or be kept hot at a minimum internal temperature of 140°F (60°C).

Buffets

Serving food buffet-style brings a unique set of challenges to food safety. Hot food must be kept hot and cold food must be kept chilled throughout the duration of the buffet. In addition, the food must be protected from contamination throughout. Any combination of failures due to time-temperature abuse and contamination by the users sets up a situation where contaminated food may be held for a number of hours at warm temperatures, allowing massive proliferation of germs. The maintenance of either hot or cold temperatures is essential for serving safe food buffet-style. More information about serving a safe buffet is given in Chapter 11.

Finger Foods

Small, individual finger foods such as canapés and sandwiches require a lot of handling during preparation and are therefore vulnerable both to contamination from the hands and to cross-contamination from other foods. Keep your hands super hygienically clean for this kind of food preparation, and keep all food preparation surfaces clean and sanitized.

Finger foods often include high-risk items such as shellfish, cooked chicken, and sauces, all of which need to be kept refrigerated as much as possible. Work in small batches, and either cook or refrigerate each batch quickly. Complete one type of finger food before starting on another, so that, for example, you are not preparing dessert items at the same time that you're working with chicken and shellfish items. When each type of food is prepared, clear everything away and clean up before starting on the next food.

Double Dipping Is a No-No

Double dipping—in reality, multiple dipping—is gross! The act of taking a chip or a vegetable stick, putting it into a dip, partially eating it, and then returning it for more dip creates a dip-saliva-germ mix. Invite or guide your guests to spoon portions of dip onto their own plates, or serve the dip in small individual containers.

13

HOME FOOD PRESERVATION

Golden Rule: Guard against botulism—the "killer in the can."

A range of food-preservation techniques can be used in the home, and there are probably thousands of recipes for everything from jams and jellies to smoked foods, to flavored oils, to canned foods. Some of the techniques are fairly simple; others are complicated and require specialized equipment. More important, some of the techniques are relatively risk-free, whereas hygiene failures in some of the techniques can lead to a very high risk of the potentially fatal illness called botulism. As mentioned earlier, the majority of cases of botulism in North America occur as a result of eating home-preserved vegetables and fish.

Recommended Reading

The USDA has produced a revised edition of its excellent reference for safe food-preservation techniques: *A Complete Guide to Home Canning, Preserving and Freezing* (Dover Publications), available at public libraries.

The purpose of this chapter is not to provide comprehensive guidelines on how to preserve food at home, but to explain both the risks involved in the different techniques and the hygiene rules that are essential in order to avoid disaster.

BOTULISM

Clostridium botulinum causes botulism. In nature, this bacteria thrives only in anaerobic environments (where the oxygen levels are low or absent), such as in the mud at the bottom of a pond or lake. But the bacteria can also survive as a dormant spore (one that will not actively grow until it finds the right conditions), and these spores can be found in the soil and on vegetables. Therefore, these spores are likely to be found on many of the raw foods that you bring into your kitchen. Most food preparation and cooking techniques kill the bacteria and the spores, thus never allowing time for the spores to grow in a low-oxygen environment. But some food-preservation techniques can create low-oxygen environments, and any *Clostridium* spores that have survived the preservation process may grow and produce the deadly botulism toxin.

Ideal conditions for the growth of *Clostridium botulinum* consist of a moist, low-acid food, a temperature between 40° and 120°F (5°–49°C), and less than 2 percent oxygen. Under these conditions, the toxin can be produced in three to four days.

The spores are resistant to heat and are difficult to destroy even at temperatures required to boil water (212°F or 100°C). Higher temperatures are achieved in canning by increasing the pressure, measured as pounds per square inch of pressure (psi). All low-acid foods should be canned in a pressure canner at 240° to 250°F (115°–121°C) and 10 to 15 psi. Low-acid foods include red meats, seafood, poultry, milk, and all fresh vegetables except for most tomatoes. Acid foods include fruits, pickles, sauerkraut, jams, jellies, marmalade, and fruit butters.

PRESERVATION TECHNIQUES

Preservation techniques can be divided into three groups: those requiring high-pressure canning, those requiring heating but not under pressure, and those requiring no heat. Although the risk of botulism is greatest for low-acid canned foods, some of the other techniques may also carry some risk for the illness.

High-Pressure Canning

High-pressure canning should be used for all low-acid foods, including meat, poultry, fish, and vegetables. Acidity is measured as pH on a scale from 1 to 14. Acid foods have a pH of 4.6 or lower, and the so-called low-acid foods have a pH higher than 4.6. Acidity can be increased by adding lemon juice, citric acid, or vinegar.

Fourteen Safety Tips

1. Carefully follow approved canning methods—do not take shortcuts.
2. Use a pressure canner with an accurate gauge, and have it tested annually.
3. Process for the full time and at the correct temperature. Follow guidelines for making adjustments for canning at higher altitudes, because water boils at lower temperatures at high altitude.
4. Use jars and lids made especially for home canning. Discard any that are cracked or nicked.

5. Never use sealing lids a second time. Once they have been processed, they never can be relied on to make a safe seal again.

6. Use firm, fresh, but not overripe vegetables. Thoroughly wash all vegetables and peel as recommended. Can as quickly as possible after harvesting—six to twelve hours for most vegetables.

7. Use only the freshest meats and poultry. Do not can meat from sickly or diseased animals.

8. Ice fish and seafood after harvest, eviscerate immediately, and can within two days.

9. Do not overpack foods—this could result in underprocessing.

10. Test each jar's seal before storing.

11. Store the processed, cooled jars in a cool, dark place, between 50° and 70°F (10°–21°C).

12. Never even taste canned foods that show signs of spoilage. Dispose of spoiled cans carefully.

13. For added safety, before serving home-canned vegetables, meat, poultry, or fish, bring them to a hard simmer (205°–210°F or 96°–99°C) for fifteen minutes.

14. Consume or dispose of all canned foods within one year.

Signs of spoilage

Contamination of canned foods with *Clostridium* is not always easy to detect, but there are some signs to watch for and which should never be ignored. *Never even taste foods from cans and jars that show any of the following signs of spoilage:*

- Signs of gas pressure, often shown by a bulging lid or by tiny bubbles in the jar that move up toward the surface
- Signs of leaking from the lid
- Any signs of damage or corrosion to the lid or jar

- An unpleasant odor when opened
- Food contents that look mushy
- Contents that have an unnatural color
- Cloudy liquid
- Any signs of mold growth

How to dispose of suspect cans

If either a home-preserved or a store-bought can or jar shows any of the above signs, then it needs to be handled as if it is contaminated with the botulism toxin and must be disposed of very carefully so that it does not contaminate anything else. If the suspect can or jar is still sealed, place it in a garbage bag, seal the bag, and place it in the regular trash or bury it in a landfill. If the suspect container is unsealed, open, or leaking, then it should be detoxified. Do this by carefully placing the container(s) and lid(s) on their sides in a large pot. Be sure to wash your hands very carefully. Add enough water to the pot to cover the jar(s) by at least an inch, and avoid any splashing. Cover the pot, and bring the water to the boiling point. Continue boiling for thirty minutes in order to destroy all traces of the toxin. When cool, discard the containers, lids, and food in the trash. Thoroughly wash any items that may have been in contact with the food or the containers, and discard all the sponges and rags used in the process in the trash.

Heating without Pressure

Fruits, pickles, and tomatoes can be safely preserved by heating the jars of these high-acid foods in a hot-water bath. The simmering hot water (180°–190°F or 82°–88°C) is enough to destroy any germs that could spoil these foods, and the high levels of acidity prevent growth of the botulism toxin.

Nine Steps to Safely Canning Fruit and Tomatoes

1. Use clean, washed equipment.
2. Discard any jars that have nicks or cracks. Use new sealing lids.
3. Scald lids in boiling water, and keep them in the hot water until ready to use.
4. Fill the boiling water bath or canner halfway with water. Preheat to 140°F (60°C) for raw-packed foods and to 180°F (82°C) for hot-packed foods.
5. When jars are in place, add more boiling water so that the water level is at least 1 inch above jar tops.
6. Bring the water to a vigorous boil, and process for the required time. Make adjustments for altitude.
7. Remove the jars and allow to cool.
8. Test each seal. Jars that have not sealed properly can be refrigerated and consumed within two days as long as there is no sign of spoilage.
9. Store jars in a cool, dark place.

Jams, Jellies, and Preserves

Jams, jellies, chutneys, and other preserves are prepared by rapidly boiling the fruit-and-sugar mixtures until they thicken. The mixtures are stored in clean, covered jars so that spoilage organisms cannot settle into them from air and dust. As a result of concerns about the possible effects of mold toxins on humans, the traditional paraffin, or wax, seals are no longer recommended for preventing mold growth on jams and jellies. Instead, the filled jars are processed for five minutes in boiling water. In the past, mold growth was simply scraped off, but mycotoxins may be left unseen in the jar (see page 81).

Use clean, washed, undamaged jars. Sterilize the jars in boiling water for fifteen minutes, and keep them immersed in the hot water until ready to use. Scald the lids in boiling water, and keep them in the hot water until ready to use. Fill the jars with the cooked fruit syrup, leaving a 1/4-inch head-space, seal with self-sealing lids, and process for a further 5 minutes in a boiling water canner or pot. Cool, label, and store in a cool, dark area.

Smoked Foods

Smoking is an ancient form of food preservation, and smoked foods are still popular today for their flavor. There are two basic methods: hot smoking and so-called cold smoking. Hot smoking uses an oven temperature up to 250°F (121°C), and cold smoking uses lower temperatures of 90° to 130°F (32°–55°C). The important thing is that the food must reach the minimum internal temperature of 160°F (70°C). Use an instant-read thermometer for this (see Chapter 10). Smoked foods must be refrigerated and eaten within four to five days, or they should be frozen. For reheating, smoked foods should reach the minimum internal temperature of 160°F.

Preserving Food without Heat

Food-preservation techniques that don't require any heating include freezing, smoking, and preparing foods such as flavored oils and pesto.

Freezing

When done correctly using high-quality fresh foods, freezing is perhaps the nearest thing to preserving food in a natural state. From a food-safety viewpoint, it's important to remember that not all food poisoning germs are killed by freezing. Some germs may survive in a state of suspended animation, and once the food is thawed, they can revive and start to multiply very quickly. That's why it's important to use the freshest high-quality raw ingredients to start with so that the germ count is low. Also, remember that any thawing that occurs allows germs to grow; therefore, it is not safe to thaw food and then refreeze it without first cooking it. Thawing and refreezing just locks in large numbers of germs into the food. Once food has thawed, it should be cooked and eaten quickly.

Flavored Oils and Pesto Sauce

Adding things like herbs and garlic to oils to give them a special flavor and making homemade pesto—a mixture of olive oil, basil, garlic, pine nuts, and Parmesan cheese—seem harmless enough. But adding fresh herbs and garlic can also carry the botulism bacteria into the oil. And as oils are both low-acid and low-oxygen and are usually not refrigerated, conditions may be just right for the growth of the germ. If you want to make flavored oils at home, look for recipes that use a cooking process to kill off the germs or that add vinegar or lemon juice to make the oil acidic, and keep these oils in the refrigerator. Oils do go cloudy in the refrigerator, but this does not spoil the flavor. Make up pesto in small batches, refrigerate it, and eat it within a few days; alternatively, make up batches for the freezer.

14

KITCHEN DESIGN AND SANITATION

> **Golden Rule:** Keep high standards of kitchen hygiene.

In many homes, the kitchen is so much more than just a place where food is served and prepared. More often than not, it's the central hub of domestic life. But some of the activities that take place in the kitchen really should not be happening in an area of food preparation and storage. Activities to do with pets, laundry, and baby care can cause the kitchen to become contaminated with the kind of germs that can cause illness.

PLANNING A KITCHEN AND CHOOSING EQUIPMENT

Whether you are planning a new kitchen for your home or simply choosing new equipment, hygiene should be one of your primary criteria. Always consider whether a surface or a piece of equipment is easy to clean, and whether access to the sink and main appliances like refrigerator, freezer, and stove is convenient. Kitchens do not have to be large and spacious in order to meet good hygiene standards, but they do need to be well organized and kept free of clutter.

111

Kitchen Counters

Kitchen counters can be made from a variety of materials, ranging from marble to stainless steel, ceramic tiles, and laminates. Surfaces that are smooth and free from gaps and cracks where dirt and germs can collect are easiest to keep hygienically clean. In this respect, ceramic tiles pose a problem because the grouting between the tiles is an area where dirt collects. Countertops should also be scratch resistant and immune to damage by bleach, detergents, and other cleaning agents.

Sinks

Sinks are usually stainless steel, enameled procelain, or plastic. Steel and procelain are the most scratch resistant and hard wearing. Again, check for the material's resistance to bleach and other chemicals. Double sinks can be advantageous, especially if you don't have a dishwasher. One sink can be used for washing kitchen utensils, and the other can be used to hold hot water for rinsing. A clear area next to the sink is needed for draining and air drying items that have been washed.

Not in the kitchen sink

Activities that should be banished from the kitchen sink include cleaning out pet tanks, emptying diaper pails, doing laundry, bathing the baby, emptying flower vases, and potting plants. If no other sink is available in an area such as a laundry room, basement, or bathroom, then use a pail of hot soapy water placed outside the kitchen or in the yard, and remember to empty the pail after each job.

Food Storage Space

A kitchen also requires some closed-off cupboard space and drawers for storing foods and utensils free from dust, pests, and pets.

Alternatively, store items on a high shelf, or hang utensils on hooks. However, utensils hanging from hooks or sitting on shelves are always exposed to dust and to grease from cooking, so they must be washed before use.

Walls and Floors

Walls and floors should be easy to clean and free from gaps and cracks where dirt can collect. A wide range of materials can be used for kitchen floors as long as it is washable. Carpeting is impossible to keep hygienically clean.

Choosing Equipment

When choosing equipment for the kitchen, especially appliances like refrigerators, mixers, slicers, and any piece of equipment in which raw food is stored and prepared, it's important to consider how easily the item can be taken apart and cleaned. Preferably, items should be safe to submerge in hot soapy water and/or be dishwasher proof.

Cutting boards

There has been a lot of discussion recently about the choice of cutting boards, and many people have strong preferences for either wooden boards or plastic boards. It has been the practice to recommend the use of hard plastic boards and to avoid the use of wooden cutting boards. This advice is based on the fact that plastic boards are less easily scratched and damaged and more easily sanitized in a dishwasher than wooden boards are. Deep scratches and gouges in any type of board can become contaminated with germs. Plastic boards are used almost exclusively in the commercial sector. But recent scientific data doesn't support the common notion that the use of wooden boards is more likely than plastics to produce cross-contamination of foods. It was also found that wooden boards can be effectively sanitized by microwaving at high setting for four minutes, whereas plastic, which is relatively inert to microwaving, cannot be sanitized successfully in the microwave. This work has undoubtedly led to some confusion and uncertainty as to what type of board to now recommend. Perhaps the best advice is still that whatever type of boards are used, they should be clean and free from deep scratches. Separate boards should be used for different foodstuffs, and all boards should be regularly cleaned and sanitized, especially after contact with raw foodstuffs. Both wooden and plastic boards can be sanitized with antibacterial kitchen cleaners or a dilution of household bleach, plastic boards can be put in the dishwasher, and wooden boards can be microwaved.

HYGIENIC HANDWASHING

Ideally, every kitchen should have a separate sink just for washing hands, but this is rarely found in domestic kitchens. The kitchen sink should be used for handwashing activities only when associated with food preparation—handwashing associated with other household jobs, gardening activities, and so forth, should be done at another sink away from the kitchen. Definitely wash your hands after using the bathroom, but do so at the bathroom sink—not at the kitchen sink.

Individual handwashing techniques vary, and some are better than others at removing germs. A good handwashing technique requires the use of soap and hot water, preferably under a running tap. Thoroughly lather the soap and rub the hands together for a count of ten to fifteen seconds, rubbing between the fingers and washing around the wrists. Then rinse under running water, and thoroughly dry the hands using a clean towel reserved for this purpose.

Bar soaps should be kept clean and should rest on a soap dish that allows water to drain away from the soap; otherwise, even bar soaps can become contaminated with germs. Pump-action dispensers for liquid soap protect the soap from contamination. Antibacterial soaps may provide some additional protection, but they do not replace the need for a thorough handwash. Antibacterial soaps are formulated to reduce bacteria on skin and should not be relied on for sanitizing hard surfaces such as countertops and cutting boards. Alcohol gels are very effective at killing microbes on the skin and can even be used in the absence of water. Both alcohol gels and antibacterial wipes are useful for traveling, camping, and picnicking.

Personal Hygiene Tips for the Kitchen

Wash hands:	Before handling food, after handling raw foods, and between handling different foods. After using the toilet, changing diapers, touching or blowing your nose, handling garbage, gardening, and handling pets.
Fingernails	Should be kept clean.
Cuts and sores on hands	Should be covered with a clean waterproof dressing.
Hair	Dry skin sheds from the scalp, carrying germs with it. Avoid brushing hair in the kitchen.

CLEANING AND SANITIZING IN THE KITCHEN

All kitchen equipment, including the refrigerator and kitchen surfaces, needs to be cleaned and sanitized, especially after contact with raw foods. Cleaning and sanitizing is usually a two-step process: step one removes any visible food, and the second step sanitizes the area. The cleaning step removes organic material, and the sanitizing step removes and kills germs, leaving a surface hygienically clean. As the name implies, antibacterial kitchen cleaners combine cleaning and sanitizing into a one-step operation, although it is still recommended that you remove food particles before applying the product.

Kitchen Equipment

Kitchen equipment should be dismantled, if possible, and all items should be run through a dishwasher cycle or submerged in hot soapy water, washed, and then rinsed in clean, hot water. Refrigerators should be regularly cleaned and sanitized using an antibacterial product. Germs can and do grow on all refrigerator surfaces.

Countertops

Countertops that have been in contact with food, especially raw food, and other areas in the kitchen that are in constant contact with hands (refrigerator handle, faucets, etc.) can be sanitized by the application of antibacterial cleaners or bleach. Use an antibacterial kitchen cleaner registered by the Environmental Protection Agency (EPA) (the registration gives assurance of an effective and approved product for food surfaces), or a dilution of household bleach or cleaning products containing bleach. The bleach should be diluted at 3/4 cup per gallon of water. Always follow manufacturer's label directions for the use of bleach and other antibacterial products. And the most hygienic practice is to use disposable paper towels in combination with antibacterial cleaners or bleach solution for wiping and cleaning kitchen surfaces.

Antibacterial Products

In the United States, antibacterial products for use on food surfaces have to pass a series of tests to show that they are both effective and safe, and then they are registered with the EPA. Many traditional home remedies, such as vinegar, lemon juice, and baking soda, have been used with the aim of killing germs on kitchen surfaces. Scientific tests have clearly shown that these home remedies cannot be relied upon to kill germs and leave surfaces hygienically clean.

Sponges and Dishcloths

Many people just take a kitchen cloth or sponge and wipe around with soapy water, but this is not good hygiene practice. Sponges and dishcloths should be kept for cleaning jobs at the sink, and the same sponge or cloth should not be used for doing other jobs around the kitchen or elsewhere. Keep separate cloths and sponges for these jobs, or better still, use paper towels. Sponges and cloths are ideal breeding grounds for bacteria, and many scientific studies have shown them to be the most heavily contaminated items in the kitchen, despite the fact that they are constantly submerged in soapy water. Even *Salmonella* can survive in sponges and cloths, and if these items are not regularly sanitized, they can be a means of spreading contamination around the kitchen. Dishcloths and sponges can be sanitized by putting them in the laundry or through a dishwasher cycle, or by submerging them in a dilute bleach solution (follow manufacturer's instructions). Moist sponges can even be sanitized by microwaving them on high power for one minute. Be careful not to microwave them for any longer than one minute, because they can burn; also, be careful when you remove them, because they get very hot in the microwave.

Ideal Breeding Ground

Sponges and dishcloths can provide the perfect living conditions for kitchen germs because they are moist and warm and often trap bits of food particles. More than 1 billion germs can grow in a sponge in twenty four hours of use.

Floors and Walls

Kitchen floors and walls can be kept clean with any general cleaning product or hot soapy water. Normally, these areas do not need to be kept hygienically clean with antibacterial or disinfectant products, because they are not in direct contact with either food or hands. An exception to this would be when there are babies and toddlers crawling on the floor. Also, in the case of accidents in which human or animal vomit, fecal material, or blood ends up on the floor, then you must take care to protect yourself from any germs while cleaning up, and you'll need to sanitize the floor.

Guidelines for Cleaning and Sanitizing in the Kitchen

Item	Cleaning/Sanitizing	How Often
All kitchen equipment and utensils	Wash in the dishwasher, or wash with hot soapy water at the sink. Air dry, or dry with a clean towel or paper towel.	After each use
Counters and contact surfaces (handles, faucets, switches, knobs, etc.)	Antibacterial kitchen cleaner or bleach and paper towel	After contact with raw food
Cutting boards	Wipe down with antibacterial cleaner or bleach, and then wash in the dishwasher or kitchen sink. Microwave wooden boards for four minutes.	After contact with raw food
Sponges	Wash in dishwasher, launder, microwave for one minute, or bleach daily. Replace regularly.	After contact with raw food
Floors and walls	Detergent product plus antibacterial products	As required

PART FIVE

SAFE COOKING FOR SPECIAL NEEDS

15

COOKING FOR HIGHER-RISK INDIVIDUALS

> **Golden Rule:** Food needs to be ultra-safe for higher-risk individuals.

As mentioned several times in this book, the term "good food" must also imply "safe food." All food that you serve at home should be safe to eat, but food needs to be even safer for some people than for others. Someone with a depressed immune system is unable to fight off infections in the same way as a person with a fully active and healthy immune system. Many people may be unaware that they are at higher risk of food poisoning (see Chapter 4). Others may know that their immune systems are depressed as a result of certain illnesses and treatments. In either case, a food poisoning infection can quickly overwhelm a depressed immune system and have extremely serious or even fatal consequences.

WHAT FOODS SHOULD HIGHER-RISK INDIVIDUALS AVOID?

Preventing food poisoning is about reducing and avoiding risk. Most of the information in this book is about reducing the risk of food poisoning through understanding the nature of food and taking appropriate actions when buying, storing, cooking, and serving it. A healthy adult with a healthy immune system may decide to make a deliberately risky eating choice—such as having a raw egg dressing for Caesar salad or eating raw oysters, sushi, and rare beef—without suffering any ill effects. But vulnerable individuals should avoid all raw foods or undercooked foods of animal origin. This may seem obvious to most people, but sometimes the food is so common and the act of eating it seems so "harmless" that they take the risk inadvertently. Typical examples: Serving undercooked hamburgers to kids—the outside of the patty looks cooked but the inside is still pink—and allowing children to taste the remains of a cookie or cake batter containing raw egg.

Higher-risk individuals need to be aware that raw foods may also be "hidden" in another food—for example, raw eggs are commonly used in desserts such as mousses, ice creams, and tiramisou, in mayonnaise, and in salad dressings such as Caesar salad, and in liquid foods such as egg nog and some so-called body-building foods.

Golden Rule: Higher-risk individuals should avoid all raw foods or undercooked foods of animal origin.

HOW TO COOK FOR A HIGHER-RISK INDIVIDUAL

If you or someone that you cook for falls into the higher-risk category, you'll need to be extra vigilant in the choice of recipes and in the practice of food hygiene from store to table (see Parts Three and Four of this book). If you are cooking for someone under medical care, ask the physician for advice.

Always shop from reputable and clean food stores, and select irradiated fresh foods if available. Choose pasteurized milk and fruit juices. Avoid soft cheeses made from unpasteurized milk. Pasteurization reduces germ counts by subjecting foods to high temperatures for a few seconds only. Never serve raw or undercooked foods of animal origin. All meats and dishes containing meat should be cooked to a minimum internal temperature of at least 160°F (70°C). And make sure that all grilled meats are thoroughly cooked. You should definitely use an instant-read thermometer to check for internal temperatures (see Chapter 10).

Always use pasteurized egg in all recipes requiring uncooked egg (ice creams, mousses, mayonnaise, etc.) and for making meringues, which are cooked at a very low temperature that may not kill all the germs. Don't serve undercooked egg dishes such as runny scrambled egg, fried egg, or soft-boiled egg, and avoid tasting cake and cookie batters containing raw egg.

Carefully rinse all fruit, vegetables, salads, and even ready-to-eat packaged salads under a running tap. Use only clean drinking water for drinks and ice cubes and for rinsing food and washing dishes.

Food Irradiation

Irradiation is a technology that would almost eliminate food poisoning germs from fresh foods, but it has not yet been fully accepted by government agencies and consumer groups in the United States. It has been approved for certain foodstuffs, including spices and some meats.

DIETARY FACTORS THAT CAN INCREASE THE RISK OF FOODBORNE ILLNESS

Perhaps the most obvious factor is the poor absorption of food, which results in people being undernourished or suffering from nutritional deficiencies. These people are at higher risk either because they are too weak to build up an adequate resistance or because they're eating poor-quality foods that often contain food poisoning germs.

The use of antacids and the consumption of contaminated fatty foods also increase the risk of food poisoning. There is some indirect evidence to suggest that drinking large volumes of water with a meal may also be a factor. Antacids change the pH of the stomach, making it easier for germs to survive. Large volumes of water dilute the acids in the stomach (making it less acidic) and also cause foods and germs to pass through the stomach rapidly, allowing less time for the acids to kill the germs. When contaminated fatty foods are consumed, the fat protects the germs from the stomach acids, and as a result, surprisingly low doses of germs may cause illness. Fatty foods that have caused illness include contaminated chocolate, cheese, and hamburgers. See Chapter 18 for more information.

Another dietary factor that can increase the risk of food poisoning is the deliberate risky eating behavior mentioned earlier. Many people enjoy raw foods of animal origin, including sushi and ceviche, clams and oysters, and undercooked beef. There are risks attached to eating all of these foods, and the risk is especially great for anyone already in a higher-risk category.

Antacids and *Salmonella*

Bill was a athletic thirty-four-year-old when he was stricken with a severe attack of *Salmonella* food poisoning. He probably got ill from eating either a chicken sandwich or an undercooked egg salad sandwich, but he'll never know for sure. His massive infection resulted in peritonitis. In an emergency operation, doctors removed four inches of Bill's colon, and he endured a temporary colostomy for the next eight months. Had it not been for Bill's great physical condition and his quick admittance to a big city hospital, he almost certainly would have died. How did Bill become so dangerously ill with *Salmonella*? Before and during the early stages of his illness, he had regularly been taking antacids.

16

COOKING FOR SENIORS AND SINGLES

People over age sixty-five are at a higher risk for food poisoning because of their aging immune systems. In addition, it is often difficult for older people to keep up with the many developments in food technology and the changing safety status of many foods. After all, if for the majority of your life, eggs have been considered a safe and nutritious food, you may find it difficult to adapt to the recent information and advice about raw and undercooked eggs. In addition to nutrition and economy, food safety also needs to be a priority for seniors.

People of any age who live alone may also find themselves inadvertently putting themselves at risk as a result of the issues surrounding cooking for one. In addition to the considerations for higher-risk groups outlined in Chapter 15, here are some additional points specifically for seniors and singles.

Shopping

Many seniors are on limited, fixed incomes and may be tempted to buy foods that are reduced in price because they are at their date-stamp limit or even beyond the limit. Selling food beyond its date limit is an illegal practice in most countries, but it still happens. These so-called bargains should be avoided, especially by seniors, because of the risk that the food is on the margins of safety. Seniors should also avoid bargain bins of dented cans and damaged packages because these foods may already be dangerously contaminated. It often makes economic sense to buy large rather than small portions of food, but doing so often results in an excess of food that has be be dealt with safely in the kitchen.

Menu Planning

Menu planning is very important for seniors and singles in order to ensure that they are eating nutritious and safe foods. It is not safe to make up a big pot of food, such as a stew or a meat sauce, and then just keep eating it over many days until it is gone. If food is cooked in bulk, it should be rapidly cooled and refrigerated to be eaten within two to three days, or cooled and immediately frozen in individual serving sizes.

Microwaving

Microwaving can be an invaluable cooking technique for seniors and singles because of the convenience of being able to cook small portions quickly and cleanly. Many people think it is too much trouble to use the oven for just one portion. Microwaving is a safe cooking technique so long as it is used correctly. It is most important that the food be cooked thoroughly and that no cold spots remain. (See Chapter 10 for more information about microwave cooking.)

Dealing with Leftovers

Chapter 11 discusses how to deal with leftovers, but that advice can present difficulties for many seniors, especially those who have long-held practices of using up leftovers, stemming from times of food shortages and the need to economize. Many people have personal family experiences of "Grandma's fridge" filled with old margarine containers, jars, and bits of plastic wrap—each containing tiny portions of leftovers, dating from who-knows-when. Leftovers should be quickly refrigerated in clean, covered containers and kept for no more than two or three days. Freezing small portions of leftovers is a better and safer idea than accumulating too many in the refrigerator. Either way, there comes a time to throw out leftovers, both for reasons of safety and because of deteriorating flavor.

Changes in the Safety Status of Traditional Foods

In addition to the changing status of their immune system, people over age sixty-five also have to come to terms with the changing safety status of traditional foods. Eggs, long held as nature's perfect food, can no longer be eaten raw or undercooked with the same level of confidence of previous years. Homemade mayonnaises are out. Raw oysters, long considered a great delicacy, can no longer be eaten raw without running the risk of dire food poisoning. Even the mainstays of chicken and beef can no longer be considered totally benign—each time you bring them into your kitchen, you need to ensure that you do not cross-contaminate other foods. And gone are all the undercooked beef recipes so beloved for so long. Because of these changes, the careful use of both refrigeration and freezing plays a much greater role in home food safety than was the case not so long ago. Many foods that were traditionally kept in a kitchen pantry must now be refrigerated, including cheeses, hams, eggs, and egg dishes such as quiches and meringues.

Home Remedies for Cleaning and Disinfection

There are many traditional home remedies for cleaning and disinfecting the kitchen, such as the use of vinegar, lemon juice, and baking soda to clean and kill germs in the refrigerator and on countertops and dishcloths. As discussed in Chapter 14, laboratory studies show that none of these traditional recipes can be relied upon as effective antibacterial treatments.

PART SIX

SAFE EATING AWAY FROM HOME

17

HOW TO AVOID FOOD POISONING À LA CARTE

Golden Rule: If in doubt, walk right out.

Eating food away from home opens a whole new area of risks and concerns, as well as pleasures and exciting eating experiences. Be it a popular upscale restaurant, a take-out, or a street vendor, wherever you eat prepared foods away from home, you put your trust in someone else's ability to serve good, tasty, fun, healthy (sometimes), quick, and *safe* food.

POINTERS TO SAFE FOOD RESTAURANTS AND TAKE-OUTS

When you eat away from home, you need to keep your eyes open and be alert to anything that will tell you whether the place you're considering is a safe place to eat, or whether you should go elsewhere. Unfortunately, there are no guarantees. Even in the most careful, hygiene-conscious establishments, things occasionally go wrong. And the superficial appearance of the place is not always the best guide. Just because a restaurant looks fancy, it doesn't necessarily mean that everything is in good shape on the other side of the kitchen door. On the other hand, well-established businesses with a good name for food know only too well that a food poisoning incident would put a big dent in their reputation, so most are very keen to avoid problems.

To be on the safe side, you might ask to be allowed to look at the kitchen. If this request is met with a negative response, you might assume that either there is something to hide back there or that they are just too busy to deal with you. If you get a No, you will have to be prepared to walk out without eating.

Visual Clues

Apart from demanding to take a tour of the kitchen, here are some small visual clues to watch for. First, any food business should be clean—floors, walls, furnishings, table linen, silverware, glasses, plates, and so on. If the place does not look clean and tidy at the customer end, it does not bode well for the kitchen either. And once you are seated at the table, don't hesitate to ask for an item to be changed because it looks dirty or chipped.

Another really good test is to check the cleanliness of the rest rooms. It's probably safer not to eat at an establishment that has dirty rest rooms. The message is that the establishment does not know the important link between food safety and good personal hygiene. Look for clean toilets, clean washbasins, plenty of soap, and plenty of paper towels or hot-air dryers.

Perhaps the biggest clue of all would be to see a member of the staff use the rest room and *not* wash his or her hands. In that case, it's time to leave, folks! Of course, the staff should always look clean and tidy. They should not have any open wounds on their hands or faces, and they should not smoke.

Also look for positive pointers such as current "safe food" awards from the local food inspector's office. These indicate that the establishment is taking part in food-safety training and inspections.

Safe Food Choices

The dangers of eating raw or undercooked foods of animal origin are discussed many times in this book. Foods such as undercooked beef and hamburgers, sushi, raw oysters, and dishes made with raw egg are currently fashionable and are on the menu in many restaurants. Healthy young adults whose immune systems are in great shape may make these risky eating choices and, most of the time, suffer no ill effects. But for anyone in the higher-risk categories for food poisoning described in Part Five, these foods are not wise choices. And if you are ordering food for your kids, remember that they, too, are at a higher risk. Ask that hamburgers be well cooked, and send them back to the kitchen if they look at all pink inside. Raw eggs are usually hidden in things like dressings, sauces, or desserts. Ask about raw eggs before you order.

Doggie Bags

Doggie bags allow you to take home all that good (and expensive) food and enjoy it later. But don't push a good idea too far. The doggie bag food is probably nearing its germ-load limit of endurance by the time you take it out of the restaurant. It's already been prepared, served, pushed around your plate, contaminated from your fork, and it has sat unchilled while you finished your coffee and made your way home. Get it into the fridge as soon as possible, and consume it within twenty-four hours. To reheat, make sure that it reaches a temperature of 160°F (70°C) or higher, or 185°F (85°C) in the microwave. If you leave the doggie bag in

the car for a few hours or overnight, don't even think of trying
to save it.

Take-Out Foods

Just like doggie bags, take-out foods may sit around for quite a
while between the time it is cooked and the time you actually eat
it. The rule is that there is a two-hour time limit from cooking to
eating or refrigerating. So, eat it, reheat it, or refrigerate it within
sixty to ninety minutes.

Street Vendors

Street vendors really operate on the outer margins of food safety,
often with even less than the minimum requirements in terms of
things like facilities for handwashing. Be very careful about the
kinds of foods that you buy from a street vendor. It's best to
buy only simple hot items that are cooked right in front of your
eyes—something you can eat immediately. Watch to make sure
that the vendor is not touching the food with his or her hands
after it's cooked.

Food Courts

In many tourist and convention cities, food courts have become
a big attraction. Many vendors are housed under one roof, and
a whole range of different ethnic foods can be bought and eaten
on the spot. As with street vendors, facilities in food courts can
be fairly basic, so be very aware of the type of food that you buy
here. Again, simple hot foods cooked in front of you are probably
the safest bet.

TRAVELING ABROAD

There are many horror stories about the terrible food poisoning illnesses that travelers endure. Almost everyone who has traveled to the underdeveloped regions of the world has a food story to relate. And it is true that the problems are more exaggerated in areas where the infrastructure is not in place to support basics like clean drinking water and sewage treatment. Before you travel, check with a travel advice organization for detailed information about the region that you intend to visit.

Don't Bring Home Unwanted Souvenirs

Many tourist resorts have sprung up in exotic parts of the world, but before paying your deposit, determine the level of development of the hotel where you're going to be staying. Fancy resort hotels in out-of-the way or primitive locations don't always have the local resources needed to support them properly. Drinking water may not be reliable, sewage treatment may be inadequate, food supplies may not be of good quality, and the staff may be lacking in food-safety training. Well-known international hotel chains may be safer bets than local "unknowns."

The advice given earlier for choosing a local place to eat at home applies wherever you go. In many countries, street vendors are best avoided altogether. Look for good standards of cleanliness and presentation in restaurants. Be very wary of the outdoor buffets that are so popular at many resort hotels. The food sits around for a long time, often in hot conditions and often exposed to flies. As a result, it can become loaded with germs. If you have a choice, select freshly prepared hot dishes, and stay away from salads and cold dishes that require a lot of handling during preparation. And don't be fooled into thinking that spicy foods will protect you from food poisoning—they don't—and the spices themselves are often contaminated with germs.

Ask about the quality of the local drinking water, and if in doubt, drink only well-known brands of bottled water. Say No to ice in your drinks if there is any concern about water quality. Oh, and don't forget about the water you use to brush your teeth—use bottled if in doubt.

EATING SAFELY AT CAMPSITES, PICNICS, AND POTLUCKS

CAMPING

Cooking at a campsite offers some extra challenges to food safety. The obvious problem is lack of refrigeration. Even on a short overnight trip, cooler space will be limited and cannot be relied on for more than about fifteen to twenty hours, depending on the air temperatures. After this time, the ice melts and the temperature inside the cooler warms up—you'll need fresh ice and a fresh supply of perishables if you plan to camp for any longer.

Planning the trip

When you are planning the food for the trip, limit the number of perishable foods, and plan to use them early in the trip. Always pack meat, poultry, fish, butter, eggs, cheese, or milk in the cooler. It's better to carry the cooler inside the car, which doesn't get as hot as the inside of the trunk. There are also plenty of foods that do not have to be kept cool—for example, canned meat and fish, canned soups and stews, condensed milk, sterilized milk, peanut butter, jelly, cereals, fruit, dehydrated foods and snacks.

The first meal

Frozen meats will slowly thaw in the cooler, ready for the first meal. Plan to cook your meat, poultry, or fish on the first night.

Remember to cook everything thoroughly and serve it hot. Check that meat and poultry is cooked until the pink is gone and there is no red in the joints. Use a bright flashlight at night so that you can see the food very clearly. In cooler weather, you can probably take bacon, eggs, lunch meat, and hot dogs to be eaten on the second day. If there are still some chunks of ice in the cooler water, then these items will still be cold enough to be safe. After the second day, be prepared to make use of canned or preserved foods if you are not able to replenish your fresh supplies.

Handwashing

It's a good idea to take along some antibacterial handiwipes or an antiseptic gel in case toilets and handwashing facilities are poor or nonexistent. Remember to wash or sanitize hands after handling raw meat and poultry and to use clean plates and utensils for the cooked food.

Drinking water

The second big challenge at a campsite kitchen is lack of clean water. Many camps do have a drinking-water tap, but if this is not available, use bottled water for drinking and cooking. Never use untreated natural water from streams, rivers, and lakes, because it is often contaminated with fecal viruses and bacteria. Natural water can be sterilized by boiling for fifteen minutes or by using commercial purification tablets (follow package directions). Allow boiled water to stand for thirty minutes so that any sediment will settle to the bottom; then, filter the water through a clean cloth.

PICNICS

Picnics and packed lunches served away from home can be hazardous, especially if they involve high-risk foods held at warm temperatures. Even in the cold of winter, hot food carried to concerts and sports stadiums can be hazardous if not kept hot enough.

Preparing and Packing a Safe Picnic

Chill all the ingredients in the refrigerator before preparation, and prepare foods as close to the time of consumption as possible. Chill foods again once they are prepared. Limit or avoid the use of high-risk foods such as shellfish, cooked meats, chicken, egg dishes, raw eggs, and cream. Choose alternatives such as spreads, peanut butter, cheeses, washed fruit, vegetables, and salads, and dried fruit and nuts. Wrap all items in food wrap or foil to protect them from contamination.

Pack picnics in insulated cool bags or boxes. Use ice or a freezer pack to maintain a low temperature. The insides of lunchboxes, coolers, and insulated totes should be wiped clean with an antibacterial cleaner or diluted bleach. If you use brown bags, use only new, clean bags. Don't re-use bags that have carried other groceries. Use antibacterial handiwipes or antiseptic gel to clean hands before handling and eating picnic food.

Kid's School Lunches

Many kids take a lunch bag to school. Because these packed lunches are not refrigerated and just sit around in hot classrooms all morning, there is plenty of opportunity for any germs in the food to multiply and create a potential for food poisoning. So, it's best not to use foods of animal origin, such as ham, chicken, salami, and egg. Instead, select safe foods such as peanut butter, hard cheeses, washed fruit and raw vegetables, dried fruits and nuts, and cookies. With a little bit of thought, kid's lunches can be nutritious and safe as well as appetizing. It's a good idea to use an insulated lunchbag with a small freezer pack. This will help to keep the food cool. Another idea is to freeze a juice box each night and add it to the lunch bag each morning. This will help to keep the bag cool, and it will be thawed by lunchtime, providing a refreshing cold drink. If you make the sandwiches the night before, wrap them and refrigerate them until morning.

Hot foods

A clean well-functioning thermos can be used to keep food hot for several hours. Rinse the thermos with boiling water, and then bring the food to as high a temperature as possible before pouring it in. Food should be kept at 140°F (60°C) or higher.

PREPARING AND COOKING FOR POTLUCKS AND NONPROFIT EVENTS

Many people volunteer to prepare and cook food at home for nonprofit events such as those held at churches and schools. This requires care because the food you prepare at home will be eaten by many people and also because the food has to be transported away from home.

Foods to Avoid

Many health departments offer guidelines on what foods to avoid for charity events at schools and other locations. These foods include baked goods that require refrigeration, legume and legume products such as chili and refried beans, meat, fish, homemade mayonnaise and cream sauces.

When to say No

Follow the guidelines presented in Chapter 12, and be sure not to take on more than you can safely handle. Keep recipes as simple as possible, and don't feel pressured to prepare and cook food if you are feeling sick.

Transporting the food

All food to be transported to a location away from your kitchen should be placed in clean containers and covered to protect the food. Foods that require refrigeration should be kept chilled and placed in a cooler for transport. Hot foods, such as thoroughly cooked casseroles, can be kept hot for transporting by insulating the casserole dish. Wrap the dish in several layers of aluminum wrap, followed by layers of newspaper and a towel. Put the wrapped casserole in the bottom of a cardboard box. To remain safe, the internal temperature of the food should be at least 140°F. Serve as soon as possible or reheat to a minimum internal temperature of 160°F. Don't reheat more than once, and discard any leftovers.

Special Permits

If the food is to be sold for profit, even at a venue such as a school, then this may require a special permit from the local health department. The local sanitary inspector may need to make an inspection, and there may be local regulations about what kinds of foods can be offered for sale. Contact the Environmental Health Division at the local public health office.

PART SEVEN

THE SCIENCE OF FOOD POISONING

18

HOW FOOD POISONING GERMS MAKE YOU ILL

Eating contaminated food does not always result in a bout of food poisoning, and those who do get ill will vary in the severity of the illness they experience. This is because several factors influence the ability of a germ or its toxin to attack the body. These include the ability of the body's defense systems to fight off the attack, the type and dose of germs taken in, and even the type of food in which the germ is hiding.

THE BODY'S DEFENSES AGAINST FOOD POISONING

The human digestive passage has its own security systems that have to be overcome before food poisoning occurs. These security systems have three levels of defense: external sensors, physical and chemical barriers, and internal attack systems.

External sensors

The eyes, nose, and mouth are the external sensors. If a food or drink looks, smells, or tastes bad or just "off," chances are that you will throw it away or spit it out rather than swallow it.

Physical and chemical barriers

The tissues lining the digestive passage act as a physical barrier to food poisoning germs entering the body. Stomach acids, deadly to many germs, act as a barrier to the movement of germs or their poisons through the system.

Internal attack systems

The body's immune system and some enzymes and bile acids present in the digestive passage zero in on invading germs to destroy them.

THE HUMAN DIGESTIVE PASSAGE

There are several ways in which food poisoning germs attack us, but the starting place for the attack is the mouth, the entrance to the human digestive passage. The human digestive passage is basically a tube that allows food to enter at one end of the body, to be turned into nutrients that the body can use, and for waste products to be expelled at the other end.

The Mouth

Food is chewed up in the mouth where it is mixed with saliva, which contains enzymes and antibodies that can destroy germs. Swallowed food is pushed through the system by wavelike muscle contractions, called peristalsis, to the stomach where it is then subjected to increasing chemical attack.

The Stomach

The stomach produces gastric juices and hydrochloric acid, which not only aids in the breakdown of food but will also kill many germs and inactivate some of their poisons, and therefore acts as a barrier to food poisoning.

The Small Intestine

Semidigested food passes into the small intestines where digestion is completed by enzymes, and nutrients are absorbed into the body. The small intestine is folded many times, but if straightened out would be about 20 feet (7 meters) long. It has a lining—the epithelium—which is very thin and which provides a surface through which nutrients can pass into the body. This process is helped further by the internal structure of the small intestine, which has extensive folds and projections (villi) in the lining that hugely increase the surface available for nutrients to be absorbed.

The small intestine has a number of defense systems of its own. These include a mechanism that collects germs and other particles in special epithelial "M" cells, where they can be attacked by the immune system. The intestine contains vast numbers of its own normal, resident bacteria—over four hundred types. Any invading bacteria has to compete with this resident population before it can become established. The ability of the normal, resident population to resist alien bacteria is greater in healthy adults than it is in young children.

Concentrated bile salts produced by the liver and that aid in the digestion of fat inhibit the growth of many bacteria that cause food poisoning. Enzymes present in the intestinal tract can attack and damage or kill many types of germs. Finally, the peristalsis that pushes food through the system may mechanically prevent bacteria from colonizing the intestines.

Should a germ penetrate the intestinal wall and escape into the body, it then has the body's immune system fighting against it.

The Large Intestine or Colon

Eventually, the semidigested food enters the large intestine, or colon, for the last 5 feet (1.5 meters) of its journey through the body. Water and electrolytes (salts of sodium and potassium) are removed, and the remaining solid waste, or feces, is expelled from the body via the rectum and anus. As much as half of the bulk of the expelled feces will be made up of bacteria.

When food poisoning occurs, the symptoms experienced depend, to some extent, on where in the digestive system the attack occurs (e.g., the stomach or the intestines) and the type of germ and its method of attack.

THE GERM

When you swallow contaminated food or drink, the type and number of germs taken in will affect your chances of getting food poisoning.

Variation in Ability to Cause Illness

The germs and their toxins that cause food poisoning are each very different in their ability to make us ill. These differences depend on the number of bacteria, viruses, or parasites that are swallowed and on the way in which they attack the body. Even different types, or species, and subtypes, or strains, of germs differ in their ability to cause illness.

Some strains of the bacteria *E. coli,* for example, produce a poison called verotoxin; others do not. Infection with a verotoxin-producing strain is more likely to develop into so-called hamburger disease, which can result in kidney failure and other serious side effects.

Some species of *Salmonella,* such as *Salmonella typhi,* are more likely to escape from the digestive passage and invade the body. So, *Salmonella typhi* infection will lead to typhoid fever, whereas infection by one of the other, more than two thousand, *Salmonella* species probably will result in a few days of diarrhea and vomiting.

The Number of Germs Needed to Cause Illness

Research has shown that the number of invading bacteria needed to cause illness can range from one to hundreds of millions. The number of organisms needed to cause infection by some of the most common food poisoning germs are given in the table below.

> Under some conditions, the dose of germs needed to cause illness may be much lower. For example, bacteria in fatty foods may better survive stomach acids.

Number of Microbes That Must Be Swallowed to Cause Illness

Microbe	Number Needed to Cause Illness
Bacteria	
Bacillus cereus	100,000–10,000,000,000
Campylobacter	500
Escherichia coli (VTEC)	1–1,000
Salmonella	1–1,000,000,000
Parasitic protozoa	1–30
Norwalk-like viruses	not known but very low

Some microbes may also be better adapted for getting into the human body and then multiplying. They do this in a number of ways, which include fooling the immune system into recognizing them as friends or by being able to resist attack by the body's defenses. *Salmonella,* for example, are not easily killed by bile acids. Most food poisoning germs attack the body in one of the four ways described next.

TYPE 1: POISON (TOXIN) PRODUCED IN THE FOOD

Staphylococcus and *Bacillus* Food Poisoning

Less than two hours after a family picnic, all six members were rushed to the hospital with severe vomiting. Four were released later the same evening, but the toddler and the grandfather needed intravenous rehydration and were kept in overnight. It took nearly three weeks for grandfather to fully recover.

Staphylococcus aureus bacteria introduced into ham sandwiches that had been made the previous day had multiplied overnight in a defective refrigerator and during the three-hour drive on a hot day to a lakeside picnic area. Incidentally, the bacteria had come from the nose of the woman who had made the sandwiches. She had touched her face several times with the same hand that she used to steady the ham as she sliced it.

This incident is typical of food poisoning caused when the bacteria *Staphylococcus aureus* multiplies on a food and produces a toxin. When the food is eaten, the toxin irritates the lining of the stomach, and the result is often severe vomiting. Because the toxin is already in the food and acts at the beginning of the digestive tract, the time between eating the food and symptoms starting—the incubation period—can be very short. Incubation periods as short as one hour have been recorded, although two to four hours is more normal. Nevertheless, it is possible to become ill before finishing a meal, if for example, this type of food poisoning happens at a dinner party.

A similar toxic food poisoning is caused by the bacteria *Bacillus cereus*. Like *Staphylococcus aureus*, the *Bacillus* bacteria produces a toxin while growing in the food. This toxin also irritates the stomach lining, resulting in vomiting, usually within one to five hours after the food was eaten. *Bacillus cereus* and related *Bacillus* species more rarely cause diarrhea.

Botulism

This very severe and potentially fatal form of food poisoning is caused by the bacteria *Clostridium botulinum*. This type of bacteria, multiplying in food in anaerobic conditions (remember, this means in the absence of air, e.g., in a canned or bottled food), produces an extremely powerful poison. A single mouthful of contaminated food has been known to result in death. Unlike the staphylococcal and bacillus toxins, the botulinum toxin passes into the bloodstream and affects the nervous system, causing symptoms within a few hours to as long as four days later, but usually within eighteen to thirty-six hours. The symptoms are tiredness, dizziness, headache, double vision, and eventually paralysis of the respiratory system and death. Fortunately, this type of food poisoning is rare, although cases occur every year in North America, usually associated with canned and bottled food and preserved meat from marine mammals. An antitoxin is available to counter the effects of the poison.

TYPE 2: POISON (TOXIN) RELEASED IN THE INTESTINES

Clostridium Food Poisoning

Unlike the Type 1 bacteria in the previous section, *Clostridium perfringens* does not produce toxin while growing in a food. When the food is eaten, the bacteria begin to form spores in what is for them the hostile environment of the intestines. It is while the cells are forming spores that they release a toxin that irritates the walls of the intestine, resulting in diarrhea.

Since the organisms have to travel further into the digestive system and because it may take a while for toxin levels to become high enough to cause illness, the incubation period tends to be longer than that of Type 1 poisoning. The incubation period is usually in the range of eight to twenty-two hours after eating the contaminated food, and symptoms of profuse diarrhea and stomach pains may last from twelve to forty-eight hours. Ill people may feel nauseous but will rarely vomit.

For example, Mrs. P. unwittingly created all the right conditions for *Clostridium perfringens* food poisoning when she prepared a favorite curry dish for her family. Her first mistake was when she decided to cook enough to last for two days. About 2 pounds of ground beef bought that morning was partially cooked in a large pot in the early evening. Spices, vegetables, and stock were then added, and cooking continued. The curry was served piping hot to the family that evening, and because the pot wouldn't fit into the refrigerator, the remainder was stored on the kitchen counter until the following evening. Warmed-up curry was served to the family about 6 P.M. the next evening. By 3 A.M. the following morning, everyone who ate the curry was ill with stomach cramps and diarrhea. Even the dog, who had eaten the leftovers, was affected. Only the baby, who had eaten canned baby food and milk, slept through the night, blissfully unaware of the competition for the bathroom.

Although usually associated with a short incubation period, *Bacillus cereus* and related *Bacillus* species can cause another, less common, diarrhea illness. This second pattern of illness results from toxin released in the intestines and typically has an incubation period of between nine and eighteen hours, followed by diarrhea for several hours.

TYPE 3: INFECTION IN THE INTESTINES

Salmonella

Salmonella is probably the best known and most common cause of food poisoning, and well over two thousand species have been identified. Commonly found on raw meat and poultry and in other foods of animal origin, these bacteria have to get past the stomach acids and into the small intestine to cause illness. Once there, the *Salmonella* bacteria will multiply rapidly, and as numbers increase, older cells begin to die off, releasing toxins. Eventually, the number of bacteria and the amount of poison increases to a point where the infected person has symptoms that include diarrhea and vomiting, fever and headache. Because this process can take some time, the incubation period can range between twelve hours and three days, but it is usually twenty to thirty-six hours.

Campylobacter

Campylobacter infection for Mr. S. meant two days of severe stomach pains and uncontrollable diarrhea, finally resulting in over a week off work. In fact, the diarrhea was so urgent that several times he soiled pajamas and sheets before he could get to the toilet. *Campylobacter jejuni,* a common cause of severe diarrhea, has an incubation period of one to ten days, although it is commonly three to five days. The main symptoms, which include severe stomach cramps and diarrhea that is often stained with bile, blood, and mucus, can last up to three days. Fever and headache may also last several days.

TYPE 4: INFECTION IN THE BLOOD AND BODY ORGANS

Miss X was in the hospital for over a hundred days before she was finally released. An illness that had started with diarrhea and vomiting the day after she ate some contaminated candy bars rapidly worsened when the *Salmonella* invaded her bloodstream and attacked internal organs. She developed abscesses on her spleen and liver, arthritis in her joints, and complications involving her kidneys. A problem with her immume system had made it easier for the *Salmonella* bacteria to pass from her digestive passage into her body and to then multiply rapidly.

Although taken in through the mouth and traveling through the digestive system, some bacteria, including *Salmonella,* can escape from the intestines and enter the blood system. Fortunately, this type of infection is relatively unusual, although it can be very serious, and the invading bacteria may attack joints such as the knees and body organs such as the kidneys, liver, heart, and brain. The reasons why this may happen relate both to the type of bacteria and to the health of the infected person. Although there may be an initial stomach upset, the main symptom is fever together with other symptoms relating to the organ(s) involved. For example, an attack on the kidneys may result in kidney failure.

Representatives of all the major groups of food poisoning organisms—bacteria, viruses, protozoa, and other parasites—can infect the human body by invading the organs. Although most *Salmonellas* rarely get beyond the lining of the intestine, a few of the two thousand types specialize in escaping into the bloodstream to cause serious illness. Probably, the best-known of these diseases is typhoid fever, which is caused by *Salmonella typhi*. Although rare in industrialized countries, typhoid is still common in nonindustrialized countries or areas where there is no properly organized disposal of human sewage. It may take as long as one to three weeks for symptoms of fever and rash to appear.

THE FOOD

The contaminated food itself, or foods eaten with it, may affect whether a person gets food poisoning or not. There are two ways in which foods can influence the chances of food poisoning occurring: by protecting the germ through the digestive system or by neutralizing some of its defense mechanisms.

Protection

A food can physically or chemically protect germs until they have passed through the stomach acid barrier and into the small intestine where the environment is more favorable for survival and growth. Foods containing a lot of fat can do this. In recent years, large outbreaks of *Salmonella* food poisoning caused by contaminated cheese, chocolate, and hamburger—all high-fat foods—have been recorded. One interesting feature of some of these outbreaks has been the very low numbers of the bacteria found in the food.

In 1982, for example, at least 272 people, mostly children, had *Salmonella* infection from eating contaminated chocolate imported into the United Kingdom from Italy. Some of the chocolate bars had fewer than twenty *Salmonella* bacteria in them, and it was only necessary to eat one chocolate bar to get ill. In this outbreak, the fat in the chocolate probably protected the small number of bacteria from stomach acids, allowing them to reach the small intestines where they could multiply and cause illness. An outbreak in the United States and Canada in the 1970s was similarly linked to chocolate containing small numbers of *Salmonella* bacteria.

Neutralizing Defenses

A food substance may temporarily neutralize the body's protective barriers. Medicines such as antacids will reduce the acidity of the stomach contents, thereby increasing the chances of a food poisoning germ reaching the intestines. Similarly, intake of large amounts of liquids with a meal, including water, may have the same effect by diluting the stomach acids and speeding up passage through the stomach.

PART EIGHT

SELF-ASSESSMENT

19

FOOD SAFETY QUIZ

TEST YOUR KNOWLEDGE OF HOW TO PREVENT FOOD POISONING

The following story is a fictionalized account of the food-handling mistakes of the Smart family, and the consequences of those mistakes. Obviously, no family could be quite as bad as Nora O. T. Smart and her husband and children, but the types of mistakes are real enough. Several examples of food poisoning scenarios occur in the lives of this invented family in a one-week period. None of the characters or situations described are based on actual people or events, and any similarity between any character and any real person, living or dead, is entirely coincidental. So, enjoy the story and use the exercise at the end to assess your own knowledge of how to handle food safely in your kitchen.

Keep a pen and paper handy, and write down all the mistakes you can find. Check your score against the answers on page 162.

The Story

As Nora's husband was being carted off to the hospital, she was sitting on the toilet trying to figure out what had gone wrong. After all, she was always so careful when it came to food. Thinking back to the previous Monday morning, she tried to recreate the week in her mind.

159

Monday had been a gloriously hot and sunny day, and with plenty of time on hand, Nora had set off in the car to the mall. Her first stop was the supermarket, where she picked up a frozen chicken and a pork loin roast, some ground beef, some stew beef, rice, and some fresh vegetables. At the checkout, Nora distributed the various foods among three or four bags, and took them out to the car. She put the bags into the trunk and hurried back to the food court, where she had arranged to meet a friend for coffee. Some two hours later, Nora finally made it home, where her first thought was to put the food away—as soon as she had checked arrangements to meet her friend again next week.

Eventually, Nora emptied the groceries onto the kitchen counter and started to put it away. She was a little surprised to find the chicken already partly defrosted and leaking bloody juices, but being a careful person, she placed it on a piece of paper towel on a plate and put it into the refrigerator on the middle shelf. "We'd better have that tomorrow," she thought to herself.

The stew beef went into the bottom of the refrigerator and the vegetables into the salad drawer. Giving the counter a quick wipe with the kitchen sponge, Nora began preparing the evening meal—chili con carne. "If I make it up now, I'll save myself time later," thought Nora. "All I'll need to do is heat it up again." She cooked the ground beef first, then later added mushroom, onion, beans, and chili sauce. The onion had been very strong, and she had several times wiped the tears off her face with her hands. Leaving the chili to cool on the stove for three hours, Nora occasionally tested the temperature with her finger before finally deciding to put it into the refrigerator.

About 5:30 P.M., Tom Smart arrived home. "We're going out for supper tonight," he announced. "I want to wind down after a hard day at work."

"But I've made chili," protested Nora.

"Leave it for the boys. They can look after themselves, and we'll go and enjoy ourselves," replied Tom.

When the boys arrived home an hour later, they found a note instructing them to cook some rice and warm up the chili. Being enthusiastic eaters, they managed to finish the lot. By 6 A.M. the following morning, both boys were suffering severe abdominal pain and diarrhea.

With two cases of diarrhea in the house, Nora was quite determined that she was going to be very careful, and strict handwashing procedures were enforced. "I'll keep things simple for the next two or three days," she thought. "The chicken had best be eaten tonight, and we can have Jell-o and ice cream."

She made a raspberry Jell-o midmorning and put it in the bottom of the refrigerator to cool and set. While she was doing this, Nora noticed that on the shelf above, the plate with the chicken was almost overflowing with bloody juices and that the piece of paper towel was completely sodden. Being a decisive person, Nora made up her mind that she would remove the chicken as soon as she had a minute and clean up the mess.

After a lunch of soup and crackers—the boys were still not eating—Nora removed the chicken, being very careful not to spill any blood, and thoroughly cleaned it in the sink by running it under lots of cold water. She patted it dry with a piece of paper towel and put it onto the counter while she searched for a roasting dish. Finally, the chicken went into the oven, and Nora could at last wipe down the counter with the kitchen sponge and have a cup of coffee. Relaxing with cup in hand, Nora noticed a small septic spot next to the fingernail on her index finger. "I must do something about that," she thought.

The roast chicken was enjoyed that evening by Nora, Tom, and their daughter, Betty. After the main meal, Nora and Tom had some Jell-o and ice cream while figure-conscious Betty ate an apple.

"I'll use the leftover chicken for your sandwiches tomorrow," Nora remarked to Betty while Tom cleared the table.

"That'll be nice," replied Betty. "But don't forget to put them in the fridge overnight. I don't want food poisoning like the boys."

Nora cleaned the remaining meat off the chicken with her fingers, then washed her hands and made the sandwiches, wrapped them in plastic, and put them in the refrigerator for the night.

The next day, barely an hour and a half after lunch, Betty suddenly rushed out of class to the bathroom where she was violently sick. In fact, she was so ill that the school principal called an ambulance, and Betty was admitted to the hospital overnight. Her worried parents were, of course, totally mystified that a second disaster had hit the family in twenty-four hours.

Later that evening, assured that Betty would survive, Nora and Tom were sitting in bed talking when Tom announced that he, too, had a queasy stomach. Within eight hours, both parents had severe diarrhea, vomiting, and fever, and Nora was left sitting on the toilet while Tom went off to the hospital. "Just a precaution," said the doctor, "since Tom has a mild heart condition."

Did You Get All the Mistakes?

1. At the store, the foods were distributed among all the bags. It would have been better to keep all the cold food together or, better still, to have put it into a cooler for transporting.
2. The food was left in the car for far too long, especially on a hot day; and even when Nora returned home, she took her time to put the food away.
3. The chicken went onto a plate that might overflow and onto a paper towel that could drip juices over the side.
4. Nora placed the chicken on the middle shelf where the meat could drip juices onto anything placed below it.
5. Nora used the kitchen sponge to wipe the counters. That sponge would get used again and become heavily contaminated. She made no attempt to sanitize the counter, the sponge, or her hands after contact with the raw foods.
6. Nora wiped her face with her hands several times while handling foods, thereby risking the transfer of *Staphylococci* from her nose.

7. She tested the temperature of the food with her finger, also risking contaminating the meat with any bacteria on her hands.

8. The chili was kept too long at room temperature, allowing *Clostridium perfringens* spores to germinate and large numbers of bacteria to accumulate in the chili. It's not surprising that the boys were ill several hours later.

9. Putting the bowl of hot Jell-o in the refrigerator would raise the temperature in the refrigerator, which would encourage bacteria to grow on other foods stored there.

10. Because the chicken was on the middle shelf, bloody juices dripped onto the raspberry Jell-o beneath. This went unnoticed because the blood blended with the color of the Jell-o.

11. Nora was always too slow to act. She did notice things, but she put off correcting potentially dangerous situations until "later."

12. Running the chicken under cold water caused splashing, which spread bacteria onto Nora's dishcloths as well as the sink surrounds.

13. Putting the chicken on the counter would contaminate this surface. Wiping the counter with the sponge would just spread the bacteria around and further contaminate the sponge.

14. As soon as Nora saw the spot on her finger, she should have covered it with a waterproof dressing.

15. Nora and Tom ate the contaminated Jell-o and just over twenty-four hours later succumbed to *Salmonella* food poisoning originating from the blood dripping from the chicken carcass.

16. Betty was right to ask her mother to put the sandwiches in the refrigerator overnight. Unfortunately, they were already contaminated with *Staphylococci* from the spot on Nora's finger as she picked the meat off the chicken carcass.

17. Contamination of the sandwiches was made worse by their being kept at room temperature in Betty's school bag all morning. By the time she ate them, there was enough toxin in the meat to make her ill very soon after lunch.
18. Not once did Nora sanitize her kitchen surfaces, and apparently she rarely washed her hands thoroughly.

How Did You Score?

If you managed to get 14 or more points, you did really well.
If you got 9 to 13 points, you have probably grasped the basics but need to brush up on some of the details.
If you got 8 points or less, you need to go back to the beginning of the book.

APPENDIX

THE ROGUES' GALLERY: AN A–Z GUIDE TO FOOD POISONING GERMS

This rogues' gallery provides a profile on each of the major causes of food poisoning—bacteria, viruses, parasites, and seafood toxins. This list includes the most common germs known to cause food poisoning. The following information is included for each:

Symptoms and incubation period
Severity of illness
Length of illness
Complications
Source of the germ
Method of spread
Foods commonly linked to illness
Safety in the kitchen

BACTERIA

Bacillus cereus

This rod-shaped bacteria causes food poisoning worldwide but is less common in the United States than in some other countries. It produces heat-resistant spores.

Symptoms and incubation period:	Produces toxins that can cause two types of illness: mainly vomiting after 1 to 6 hours; mainly diarrhea after 6 to 24 hours.

Severity of illness: Generally illness is relatively mild
                              and self-limiting.

Length of illness: It is unusual for the illness to last
                              longer than 24 hours.

Complications: None usually.

Source of the germ: Widespread in the environment, in
                              soil and dust, and is common on
                              raw and dried foods.

Method of spread: Spores that survive cooking will
                              germinate in food stored at room
                              temperature. Spores found on
                              raw cereals and vegetables and
                              on dust.

Foods commonly   Cereals, especially rice; vegetables
  linked to illness: and spices; pasta.

Safety in the kitchen

Temperature control of foods that are not to be eaten immediately
after cooking is very important. Leftovers should be cooled as
soon as possible and kept refrigerated. Reheated food should be
quickly heated to 160°F (70°C) and eaten right away. If possible,
avoid making up more food than is needed for one sitting. Keep
kitchen surfaces and equipment clean.

Brucella abortus (Brucellosis)

A small bacteria that ranges in shape from rounded to rod-shaped.
Found worldwide but particularly in Mediterranean countries, the
Middle East, Asia, and Central and South America. Now unusual
in countries that have eradicated brucellosis in animals. The bacteria are killed by pasteurization. A related bacteria, *Brucella melitensis,* causes a similar illness.

Symptoms and incubation period:	Escapes into the body, causing fever, headache, sweating, joint pain, weight loss, and depression; localized infections can occur. Fever may come and go. Onset after exposure is usually 1 to 8 weeks.
Severity of illness:	Can be severe with complications.
Length of illness:	From a week to a year or longer if not properly treated.
Complications:	Abscesses on internal organs; damage to arteries, joints, heart, and testes. Death in about 2 of every 100 untreated cases.
Source of the germ:	Cattle, pigs, goats, sheep, wild elk, deer, caribou, bison, and coyotes.
Method of spread:	By contact with infected body fluids and tissues, particularly the placenta. Drinking contaminated milk and dairy produce.
Foods commonly linked to illness:	Raw milk from cows, goats, and sheep. Cheese and other dairy products made from raw milk.

Safety in the kitchen

Avoid raw milk and raw milk cheeses, particularly in the regions named above.

Campylobacter jejuni

A common cause of diarrhea worldwide, especially in children. It grows best at just above body temperature but is killed by pasteurization and normal cooking temperatures. As many as 2 million cases of diarrhea a year in the United States.

Symptoms and incubation period:	Mild to severe illness is marked by diarrhea, stomach pains, fever, and nausea, but vomiting is less common. Blood may be seen in feces. Symptoms start 1 to 10 days after swallowing the germ.
Severity of illness:	Mild to severe and may last longer in adults. Rare complications.
Length of illness:	Usually 2 to 5 days and rarely more than 10 days. Relapses can occur.
Complications:	Arthritis, Guillain-Barré syndrome, or meningitis. Can mimic appendicitis.
Source of the germ:	Cattle, poultry, and other animals, including puppies and kittens. Raw poultry meat is frequently contaminated.
Method of spread:	Eating contaminated foods, either raw or undercooked, and drinking contaminated water. Contact with infected animals, particularly pets.
Foods commonly linked to illness:	Poultry meat, beef, pork, shellfish, and unpasteurized milk. Nonchlorinated water, also.

Safety in the kitchen

Contaminated poultry may be an important vehicle for bringing *Campylobacter* into the kitchen and contaminating other surfaces. Keep raw meat, including poultry, away from other foods, and sanitize work surfaces after contact with raw meat. Wash hands after handling raw meat, and do not put hands to the mouth while handling raw meat. Avoid drinking or eating while handling raw meat. Keep pets away from kitchen work surfaces, and wash hands after touching pets.

Clostridium botulinum (Botulism)

This rod-shaped bacteria produces a dangerous poison in food that attacks the nervous system, resulting in paralysis and, sometimes, death. Cases occur worldwide.

Symptoms and incubation period:	The initial symptoms, blurred or double vision, difficulty in swallowing, and dry mouth usually occur within 12 to 36 hours but can take up to a week. Vomiting, diarrhea, or constipation are some early symptoms. Late symptoms include paralysis.
Severity of illness:	Symptoms are severe. Death occurs in about 5 to 10 of every 100 people who are reported to have botulism.
Length of illness:	Recovery can take many months.
Complications:	Prolonged recovery period.
Source of the germ:	Bacterial spores are found everywhere; in the soil and in the digestive passage of some animals and birds.
Method of spread:	Eating food in which growing cells have already produced toxin; improperly canned and bottled products are a particular risk.
Foods commonly linked to illness:	Improperly canned and bottled products, especially those prepared in the home; seal meat and smoked salmon, sausages and smoked preserved meat. Some vegetables.

Safety in the kitchen

Careful home canning and bottling procedures to ensure adequate heating for the correct length of time. Discard any cans (commercial or home-produced) that show signs of damage or dents.

Clostridium perfringens

Related to *Clostridium botulinum,* this rod-shaped bacteria causes food poisoning worldwide.

Symptoms and incubation period:	Usually causes mild diarrhea and nausea, but rarely vomiting, within 6 to 24 hours of eating.
Severity of illness:	Most people get a fairly mild illness.
Length of illness:	Usually less than one day.
Complications:	Usually none, but has caused a severe form of enteritis with higher-than-normal death rates. Deaths are otherwise rare.
Source of the germ:	Found in the soil and the digestive tract of animals such as cattle, pigs, poultry, and fish.
Method of spread:	Eating food contaminated by soil or feces in conditions that allow multiplication of the bacteria.
Foods commonly linked to illness:	Usually meat stews, casseroles, pies, and gravies not cooked properly or inadequately reheated.

Safety in the kitchen

Keep control of temperatures in kitchen and refrigerator—that is, keep hot foods very hot or cold foods very cold. Do not reheat food more than once.

Cyclospora cayetanensis

This newly recognized diarrheal disease has been particularly linked to eating raw soft fruits and is caused by a protozoa-like parasite.

Symptoms and incubation period:
: Watery diarrhea with nausea, stomach pains, fatigue, loss of weight and appetite.

Severity of illness:
: From mild to severe with diarrhea lasting up to 6 weeks.

Length of illness:
: Self-limited but may last several days in healthy people.

Complications:
: Diarrhea can last for months in people with depressed immunity.

Source of the germ:
: Usually water contaminated with feces.

Method of spread:
: Mainly through drinking or swimming in contaminated water, or eating foods that have been in contact with contaminated water.

Foods commonly linked to illness:
: Illness has been linked to eating soft fruit and vegetables that may have been washed or irrigated with contaminated water.

Safety in the kitchen

Special care in personal hygiene for infected people, who should also avoid handling foods that are not to be cooked before eating. Special care should be taken to avoid drinking untreated water, particularly in nonindustrialized regions.

Escherichia coli (Hamburger Disease)

Rod-shaped bacteria that produce verotoxins. First recognized after an outbreak in the United States in 1982, *E. coli*

has been called hamburger disease because a number of outbreaks have been traced back to hamburgers. Outbreaks have
been reported in the United States, Canada, Europe, South Africa,
Japan, and Australia.

Symptoms and incubation period:	Symptoms can occur 3 to 8 days after exposure and include mild diarrhea to severe diarrhea with a lot of blood.
Severity of illness:	Mild to severe illness leading to kidney failure and death.
Length of illness:	Varies with severity from a few days to many weeks. Longer if complications occur.
Complications:	Breakdown of red blood cells and impaired kidney function, sometimes leading to temporary or even permanent kidney failure.
Source of the germ:	Appears to be mainly cattle, although infected people can also pass it on.
Method of spread:	Usually by eating contaminated food or drinking water, or directly from person to person.
Foods commonly linked to illness:	Inadequately cooked ground beef products such as hamburgers and raw milk. Potentially any food contaminated with cow manure.

Safety in the kitchen

Cook beef thoroughly, especially hamburgers, until no pink color
is visible in the center. Wash hands and surfaces well, and then
disinfect counters.

Listeria monocytogenes (Listeriosis)

A rod-shaped bacteria that can be transmitted in food, although rarely. Unborn babies, elderly people, and others with depressed immunity are at particular risk of serious illness.

Symptoms and incubation period:	May range from a mild flu-like illness to inflammation of brain tissues. Headache, fever, nausea, and vomiting. Can affect the heart and other internal organs. In most cases, illness occurs 3 weeks after infection.
Severity of illness:	Can be very serious and lead to death, although symptomless infections have been recorded.
Length of illness:	Varies with severity.
Complications:	Can affect the heart and cause internal abscesses, meningitis, septicemia, and abortion. People with depressed immunity, including pregnant women, are at particular risk of serious illness.
Source of the germ:	Environment; soil, water, silage. Some domestic and wild animals.
Method of spread:	Contaminated food. From infected mother to unborn baby.
Food commonly linked to illness:	Contaminated raw milk, soft cheeses, pâté, and contaminated vegetables.

Safety in the kitchen

Limit cross-contamination in the kitchen by practicing good hygiene. Thoroughly wash fresh vegetables, salads, and prepackaged salads before use.

Salmonella (2,000 types)

These rod-shaped bacteria are a major cause of food poisoning worldwide. They are commonly found in animal intestines, and animal feces may contaminate food and water. They multiply rapidly at body temperature but are readily killed by pasteurization and by cooking. More than two thousand aliases (serotypes) are known, but most illness is caused by only a few hundred types.

Symptoms and incubation period:	Diarrhea, vomiting, and fever usually from 6 to 72 hours after swallowing.
Severity of illness:	Mild to severe. Deaths occasionally, particularly in the very young, very old, those with existing serious illness, and the immunocompromised.
Length of illness:	From 1 to 7 days. Some people may excrete for weeks even after symptoms have stopped.
Complications:	Blood poisoning, meningitis, and bone-joint infections most often.
Source of the germ:	Human and animal feces. Human cases have been associated with infected pets, such as turtles, terrapins, hedgehogs, dogs, and cats.
Method of spread:	Contaminated food and water. Less often from person to person.
Foods commonly linked to illness:	Poultry and other meats, eggs, and milk. However, a wide variety of foods as diverse as chocolate and bean sprouts have been linked to illness.

Safety in the kitchen

Prevent cross-contamination in the kitchen, and ensure that food is cooked thoroughly to destroy all *Salmonella*. Do not give *Salmonella* the chance to multiply by leaving risk foods at room temperature too long.

Salmonella typhi and *S. paratyphi* (Typhoid)

Typhoid (and paratyphoid) is caused by a *Salmonella* that specializes in escaping from the intestines and invading the body. Although it is found worldwide, it occurs most frequently where there is poor sanitation.

Symptoms and incubation period:	Symptoms may begin 1 to 4 weeks after infection and include fever, a general feeling of illness, severe headache, loss of appetite and sometimes spots on the body. Constipation is more common than diarrhea.
Severity of illness:	Generally more severe than other *Salmonella*, although paratyphoid is usually milder. Up to 1 in 10 cases are fatal if not treated.
Length of illness:	Can last weeks to months, and some people (carriers) can carry the bacteria in their intestines for months or years without symptoms.
Complications:	Intestinal hemorrhage or perforation. Relapses in some cases.
Source of the germ:	Humans are the main source of typhoid and paratyphoid bacteria.
Method of spread:	Food and water contaminated by human feces and urine. Hands of carriers.

Foods commonly   Will vary with the country, but
  linked to illness: potentially includes any fresh fruit or
                          vegetables irrigated or fertilized with
                          feces-contaminated water. Impure
                          drinking water. Shellfish harvested
                          from sewage-contaminated water.

Safety in the kitchen

Special care in handwashing and personal hygiene. Thorough
washing of all raw fruits and vegetables (this may not remove all
bacteria) using boiled or treated water.

Shigella (Shigellosis)

Food poisoning by this rod-shaped bacteria occurs through contamination with feces. It occurs worldwide and spreads rapidly from
person to person, especially in situations of poor personal hygiene.

Symptoms and   Diarrhea, fever, nausea, vomiting, and
  incubation period: stomach cramps usually starting up to
                          a week after exposure. Blood and
                          mucus may be seen in feces.
Severity of illness: Varies with age, nutritional status, and
                          type of *Shigella* (there are four main
                          types, or species). An important cause
                          of death in children in areas of poor
                          nutrition. Symptomless infection can
                          occur.
Length of illness: Most people get better in 4 to 7 days in
                          uncomplicated infections.
Complications: Convulsions in young children. Produces
                          a similar poison (toxin) to hamburger
                          disease, resulting in possible kidney
                          failure.

Source of the germ: Humans.
Method of spread: By consuming food or drink contaminated with feces, and from person to person.
Foods commonly linked to illness: Any food or drink that is contaminated with feces.

Safety in the kitchen

Very high standards of personal hygiene to prevent spread to food. Special care with handwashing.

Staphylococcus aureus

This ball-shaped bacteria causes an estimated 1.5 million cases of food poisoning in the United States annually. Staphylococci make a heat-resistant poison, able to survive boiling for thirty minutes, in the food before it is eaten.

Symptoms and incubation period: Vomiting can start as quickly as 1 to 6 hours after eating food containing the poison.
Severity of illness: Symptoms can be very intense, resulting in admission to a hospital, although death is rare.
Length of illness: Usually 1 to 2 days and less commonly several days.
Complications: Complications or death are rare.
Source of the germ: Often in the nose and throat and on the skin of healthy individuals and in septic spots and cuts. Raw milk from cows with udder infections.
Method of spread: Bacteria from a septic spot or infected nasal secretion may be readily transferred to a food by handling.

Foods commonly   Foods that require a lot of handling in
   linked to illness: their preparation, such as sandwiches,
                            pastries, cold meats, salty meats.

Safety in the kitchen

It is very important to minimize touching of foods and to ensure
that cuts, spots, boils, and sores are covered with a waterproof dressing. Do not allow foods to stand at room temperature for any length of time; keep hot foods piping hot and cold
foods cold. Once the poison is made, it may not be destroyed
by cooking.

Vibrio cholerae O1 (Epidemic Cholera)

Unlike other vibrio bacteria, epidemic cholera is linked to large
community-wide outbreaks. Found in Asia and Africa, and since
the early 1990s has caused widespread illness in South
America.

Symptoms and   Characteristic acute onset of profuse
   incubation period: watery diarrhea 1 to 3 days after
                            infection. If not treated, profuse
                            diarrhea causes rapid dehydration
                            resulting in kidney failure.
Severity of illness: Often severe, and can result in death
                            if not treated.
Length of illness: Up to several days.
Complications: Renal failure and circulatory collapse.
Source of the germ: Humans and brackish water
                            environments.
Method of spread: By ingestion of food contaminated by
                            feces-contaminated water.

| Foods commonly linked to illness: | Contaminated drinking water, raw or undercooked seafood. Raw fruit and vegetables washed with contaminated water. |

Safety in the kitchen

Special care in personal and kitchen hygiene, especially when preparing seafood. Thorough cooking of seafood.

Vibrio parahaemolyticus

A curved, almost comma-shaped bacteria that is found in many parts of the world, including the United States and Asia. This bacteria is one of the commonest causes of food poisoning in Japan.

Symptoms and incubation period:	Watery diarrhea usually starts about 12 to 14 hours after infection but can be up to 3 days, and is accompanied by stomach cramps and sometimes nausea, vomiting, fever, and headache.
Severity of illness:	Usually mild to moderate and is self-limiting.
Length of illness:	Up to a week.
Complications:	Rarely invades the body or causes death.
Source of the germ:	Naturally found in seawater and seabed silt. Seafood.
Method of spread:	Consumption of raw or partially cooked seafood. Cross-contamination from seafood or sea water.
Foods commonly linked to illness:	Raw and undercooked seafood.

Safety in the kitchen

Special care in kitchen hygiene to avoid cross-contamination. Cook seafoods for at least 15 minutes at 160°F. Other noncholera vibrios cause a similar illness that is also linked to seafood.

Vibrio vulnificus

Another vibrio bacteria. Can cause serious illness in certain groups of people.

Symptoms and incubation period:	Illness can start as early as 12 hours and as long as 3 days after infection. Invades the blood, causing serious illness in persons with liver disease, blood disorders, or depressed immunity.
Severity of illness:	Severe and a high death rate in groups mentioned above.
Length of illness:	May last from days to weeks.
Complications:	Blood clotting irregularities.
Source of the germ:	Marine environment.
Method of spread:	Eating contaminated seafood.
Foods commonly linked to illness:	Seafood, especially shellfish such as raw oysters.

Safety in the kitchen

High standards of personal and kitchen hygiene. Raw seafood should be avoided by those at higher risk of serious illness.

Yersinia enterocolitica

A rod-shaped bacteria found worldwide. A high proportion of reported cases occur in young children.

Symptoms and incubation period:	Usually symptoms start 1 to 7 days after infection. Symptoms include acute diarrhea and fever and appendicitis-like pains (this infection can be mistaken for appendicitis). Bloody diarrhea is seen in up to a third of child cases. About half of adults experience painful joints.
Severity of illness:	Mild to moderate illness that is usually self-limiting.
Length of illness:	From days to weeks if there are complications.
Complications:	These include arthritis-like symptoms and internal infection of the blood and body organs.
Source of the germ:	Animals, pigs particularly.
Method of spread:	Consumption of food or water contaminated with animal feces.
Foods commonly linked to illness:	Pork, milk and milk products.

Safety in the kitchen

High standards of kitchen hygiene, including handwashing, to avoid cross-contamination from raw meat. Avoid consumption of raw pork and unpasteurized milk.

VIRUSES

Hepatitis A

This virus infection is reported worldwide and is common in children where sanitation is poor. Cooking temperatures of 194°F (90°C) or over destroy the virus. Periodic epidemics have been recorded in the United States, peaking in 1961, 1971, and 1989, and outbreaks linked to food occur.

Symptoms and incubation period:	The time between infection and onset of symptoms is usually 4 to 6 weeks. Symptoms include fever, feeling unwell, no appetite, nausea, followed after a few days by jaundice (skin and eyes take on a yellowish tinge).
Severity of illness:	Usually a fairly mild illness, but rare, very severe cases occur. Severity increases with age.
Length of illness:	Weeks to months depending on severity.
Complications:	Rare severe illness lasting several months.
Source of the germ:	Humans. Large numbers of viruses may be excreted in feces.
Method of spread:	Fecal-oral transmission from person to person as well as via sewage-contaminated water and food.
Foods commonly linked to illness:	Shellfish harvested from sewage-contaminated water, and contaminated raw fruit and vegetables.

Safety in the kitchen

Care in personal and kitchen hygiene with special attention to handwashing. Shellfish should be steamed for a minimum of ninety seconds.

Norwalk-like Viruses

Named after the town of Norwalk, Ohio, this group of related viruses cause gastroenteritis worldwide.

Symptoms and incubation period:	Illness is usually characterized by acute onset of diarrhea, nausea and vomiting, stomach pains, headache and mild fever 24 to 48 hours after infection.
Severity of illness:	Usually a mild to moderate self-limited illness.
Length of illness:	Symptoms generally last 24 to 48 hours, although a small proportion of cases may feel unwell for several days.
Complications:	None usually.
Source of the germ:	Human feces.
Method of spread:	Generally, feces-contaminated food, particularly shellfish, and water. Possibly also airborne and via contact with surfaces contaminated with feces and vomit, even if this cannot be seen.
Foods commonly linked to illness:	Mollusks and any seafood that may have been contaminated with sewage or sewage-polluted water.

Safety in the kitchen

Cooking of raw shellfish for a minimum of four minutes at 194°F. High standards of hygiene, particularly when a member of the household is ill with diarrhea and vomiting.

PARASITES

Cyclospora cayetanensis

This newly recognized diarrheal disease has been particularly linked to eating raw soft fruits and is caused by a protozoa-like parasite.

Symptoms and incubation period:	Watery diarrhea with nausea, stomach pains, fatigue, loss of weight and appetite.
Severity of illness:	From mild to severe with diarrhea lasting up to 6 weeks.
Length of illness:	Self-limited but may last several days in healthy people.
Complications:	Diarrhea can last for months in people with depressed immunity.
Source of germ:	Usually water contaminated with feces.
Method of spread:	Mainly through swimming in or drinking contaminated water. Eating foods that have come in contact with contaminated water.
Foods commonly linked to illness:	Illness has been linked to eating soft fruit and vegetables that may have been washed or irrigated with contaminated water.

Safety in the kitchen

Special care in personal hygiene for infected people, who should also avoid handling foods that are not to be cooked before eating. Special care to avoid drinking untreated water in nonindustrialized regions in particular.

Cryptosporidium parvum (Cryptosporidiosis)

This tiny, single-celled protozoa-like parasite has become recognized as an important cause of diarrhea worldwide in recent years. The parasite can survive normal chlorination of drinking water.

Symptoms and incubation period:	A mainly diarrhea illness starting 1 to 2 weeks after infection, may also include stomach pains, fever, nausea, and vomiting. Symptoms may come and go for several weeks.
Severity of illness:	From very mild to very severe.
Length of illness:	Usually up to 3 weeks.
Complications:	Can cause serious illness and death in people with depressed immunity, including AIDS patients.
Source of germ:	Mainly feces of humans and domesticated animals.
Method of spread:	Fecal-oral route, including person to person, waterborne and foodborne routes. Water sources may be contaminated by rainwater runoff from grazing lands.
Foods commonly linked to illness:	Illness has been linked to drinking contaminated water.

Safety in the kitchen

Special care in personal hygiene. Infected persons should avoid handling foods that are not to be cooked before eating. In risk areas, drinking water should be boiled for at least one minute before cooling and use.

Giardia lamblia (Giardiasis)

Another single-celled protozoa-like parasite that has a worldwide distribution. Infection is associated with poor sanitation and poor hygiene, particularly in care facilities for young children.

Symptoms and incubation period:	Illness may take from 5 days to 3 weeks to develop and can result in diarrhea, stomach cramps, bloating, fatigue, and loss of weight. Feces may be pale and greasy looking.
Severity of illness:	Varies from mild to moderately severe. Many people have unnoticed infections.
Length of illness:	Recovery can take from weeks to months.
Complications:	Can cause arthritis and severe infection, may damage parts of the digestive tract.
Source of germ:	People and some domestic and wild animals.
Method of spread:	Fecal-oral transmission from person to person, by transferring the microbe from hand to mouth, is probably the most common method of spread. Waterborne outbreaks have occurred, resulting from contamination of a water source by, for example, water runoff from grazing land. Water treatment with chlorine may not kill off the cysts of *Giardia*.
Foods commonly linked to illness:	Contaminated water.

Safety in the kitchen

High standards of personal hygiene, especially handwashing. Contaminated drinking water should be boiled.

Trichinella spiralis (Trichinosis)

Illness is caused by a parasitic worm that makes its home in the intestines. The larvae, however, migrate into the body and lodge in the muscles. Although worldwide, occurrence of illness is usually linked to eating undercooked pork and horse meat and meat from wild animals. Unusual in the United States at the present time, although single cases and occasional local outbreaks are reported.

Symptoms and incubation period:	Illness can start between 1 and 7 weeks after eating contaminated food. Diarrhea and fever may be the first symptoms; illness is characterized by sore and painful muscles and swollen eyelids. Later symptoms include pain and hemorrhages in the eyes, thirst, chills, sweating, and weakness.
Severity of illness:	Varies from very mild to serious fatal illness.
Length of illness:	Weeks to months.
Complications:	Heart and neurological complications occur in severe cases and can lead to heart failure and death.
Source of germ:	Pigs, horses, cats, and dogs and many types of wild animals, including marine mammals, can harbor this parasite.

Method of spread: Consumption of undercooked meat:
                          pork, horse, and many wild animals.
Foods commonly   Pork, horse meat, and meat of many
   linked to illness: wild animals.

Safety in the kitchen

Thorough cooking of all pork and pork products and other
risky meats. When cooked, the meat should be gray, with no
pink visible.

SEAFOOD TOXINS

A number of toxins have been linked to seafood, both fish and
shellfish. These toxins may be products of the breakdown of fish
flesh (Scombrotoxin), the products of plankton growing in the
water from which shellfish were harvested (Paralytic Shellfish Poison), and toxins naturally present in the fish or shellfish (Tetrodotoxin). The most common are described below; many act on the
nervous system.

Scombrotoxin: Rapid onset of an allergic-type
                          reaction that can vary in severity.
                          Particularly linked to mackerel,
                          tuna, bluefish, and others.
Paralytic Shellfish   Plankton produce toxins that affect
   Poisoning (PSP):   the nervous system. Severe
                          poisoning can result in death.
                          Shellfish are the source of human
                          illness.
Diarrhetic Shellfish   Another toxin produced by plankton,
   Poisoning (DSP):   this one causing diarrhea. Illness is
                          associated with mollusks such as
                          clams, mussels, and oysters.

Neurotoxic Shellfish Poisoning:	This plankton-produced toxin attacks the nervous system. The toxin can be accumulated by mollusks.
Domoic Acid:	This plankton-produced toxin causes mild to very severe illness characterized by loss of memory. Associated with mollusks.
Ciguatoxins:	This poison causes a mix of symptoms resulting in gastrointestinal symptoms and neurological problems. The symptoms are caused by toxins that accumulate in fish that feed on certain plankton.
Tetrodotoxin:	A powerful neurotoxin concentrated in the skin and viscera of puffer fish, porcupine fish, and sunfish. The death rate may be as high as 60 of every 100 people affected.

GLOSSARY

Aerobic
The presence of oxygen in a usable state.

Anaerobic
The absence of oxygen in a usable state.

Antibacterial cleaner
A product that is formulated both to kill bacteria and to clean surfaces.

Bacteria
Simple microbes that multiply by dividing in two.

Bug
See *Germ*.

Clean
To remove grease and organic particles such as food.

Contaminant
Any substance, object, or germ that has found its way into the food but that should not normally be there.

Cross-contamination
The transfer of germs or chemicals from one surface to another.

Dehydration
The loss of essential body fluids and chemicals, particularly sodium and potassium.

Detergents
A mixture of soap and other synthetic substitutes used in cleaning to remove grease and other dirt.

Enteric infections
Infections of the digestive system.

Food poisoning   Any illness that results from consuming a harmful food. This can be caused by substances naturally found in the food or by contaminating chemicals or germs.

Foodborne dysentery Acute diarrhea caused by pathogens in food.

Fungi   Mushrooms, molds, and yeasts—some of which can cause illness.

Gastroenteritis   An inflammation of the stomach and intestinal tract that normally results in diarrhea.

Germ   A term commonly used to describe the bacteria, viruses, protozoa, and parasites that cause illness.

Histamine   A chemical released by cells that causes allergy-like symptoms.

Immunity   The body's natural ability to resist infection.

Incubation period The time between exposure to a pathogen or toxin and the onset of symptoms.

Microbe   Tiny lifeforms that are generally visible only through a microscope; e.g., bacteria, viruses, protozoa, and some parasites.

Mycotoxins   Toxins produced by fungi.

Offal   The internal organs and soft tissue that are removed from a carcass when an animal is butchered.

Parasite   In this book, the term refers to worms and protozoa. In its wider context, it includes bacteria, viruses, fungi, and any creature that lives on or in another.

Pasteurization   A process for treating milk and other foods at a specific temperature and for a specific time in order to destroy pathogenic germs.

Pathogen   A microbe that causes illness.

Phage type   A subdivision within a species of bacteria that depends on whether a bacterial cell is killed by certain viruses called bacteriophages. These viruses specifically attack bacteria.

Plankton   Tiny plants and animals that tend to be free-floating in fresh water and seawater.

Protozoa   Single-celled animals found in soil and water.

Refrigeration   Keeping food at a temperature above freezing but below 40°F.

Sanitize   To kill and/or remove germs to safe levels from surfaces such as counters and cutting boards.

Shelf life

The length of time in which a processed food remains safe, as determined by the manufacturer and noted on the label.

Species

A group of organisms that are very closely related will belong to the same species. Members of the group will have specific names; e.g., *Bacillus* species include the members *Bacillus cereus* and *Bacillus subtilis*. Tests can differentiate subspecies, subtypes, and strains within a species.

Spore

A dormant state in bacteria that protects genetic and other materials needed for life from the environment. They are often very resistant to extremes of temperature, dehydration, and chemical action.

Sterilization

A process that destroys all microbes.

Strain

A variant of a species member.

Symptoms

The physical manifestations of illness.

Toxins

Poisons produced by pathogenic bacteria.

Verotoxins

Powerful toxins produced by some subtypes of *E. coli*.

Virus

Microbes that are smaller than bacteria and that need to use a host cell to replicate.

BIBLIOGRAPHY

"Australia's Notifiable Diseases Status, 1996." *Communicable Disease Intelligence* 21 (1997): 281–310.

Benenson, Abram S., ed. *Control of Communicable Diseases in Man Manual*, 16th edition. Washington, DC: American Public Health Association, 1995.

Buzby, J. C., T. Roberts, C.-T. Jordan-Lin, and J. M. MacDonald. *Bacterial Foodborne Disease: Medical Costs and Productivity Losses*. Food and Consumer Economics Division, Economic Research Service, U.S. Department of Agriculture. Agriculture Economic Report No. 741, 1996.

Cohen, F. L., and D. Tartesky. "Microbial Resistance to Drug Therapy: A Review." *American Journal of Infection Control* 25 (1997): 51–64.

A Complete Guide to Home Canning, Preserving and Freezing. USDA Revised edition. New York: Dover, 1994.

Council for Agricultural Science and Technology. *Foodborne Pathogens: Risks and Consequences*. Task Force Report No. 122. AMES IA CAST 1994.

Dimblebey, Josceline. *The Cook's Companion*. London: Sainsbury, 1991.

The Food and Drink Federation and the Institution of Environmental Health Officers. *National Food Safety Report*. London: The Food and Drink Federation, 1993.

The Food Safety (General Food Hygiene) Regulations (UK)-S.I. No. 1763 Department of Health, London: HMSO, 1995.

Fox, Nicols. *Spoiled—The Dangerous Truth about a Food Chain Gone Haywire*. New York: Basic Books, 1997.

Hobbs B. C., and D. Roberts. *Food Poisoning and Food Hygiene* (5th edition). London: Edward Arnold, 1987.

Lehmann, Robert H. *Cooking for Life: A Guide to Nutrition and Food Safety for the HIV-positive Community*. New York: Dell, 1997.

Ministry of Agriculture, Fisheries and Food (UK). *Food Hygiene: Report on a Consumer Survey*. London: Her Majesty's Stationery Office, 1988.

Nagle, Mary. "When Good Foods Go Bad," *Prevention*, August 1997, 86–95.

Parmley, Mary Ann. *Safe Food to Go: A Guide to Packing Lunches, Picnicking and Camping Out*. Washington, DC: USDA Food Safety and Inspection Service, 1985.

Report of the American Society of Microbiology Task Force on Antibiotic Resistance. Supplement to: Antimicrobial Agents and Chemotherapy. American Society for Microbiology, Washington, DC, 1995.

Scott, Elizabeth. "Food Safety in the Home." In *Safe Handling of Foods*, edited by J. M. Farber and E. C. D. Todd. New York: Marcel Dekker. In press.

Scott, Elizabeth. "A Review of Foodborne Disease and Other Hygiene Issues in the Home." *Journal of Applied Bacteriology* 80 (1996): 5–9.

Serving Safe Food. A Practical Approach to Food Safety. Certification Cookbook. Chicago: The Educational Foundation of the National Restaurant Association. 1995.

Sockett, P. N. "The Epidemiology and Cost of Diseases of Public Health Significance, in Relation to Meat and Meat Products." *Journal of Food Safety* 15 (1995): 91–112.

Sockett, Paul. "Social and Economic Aspects of Foodborne Disease." *Food Policy* 18 (1993): 110–119.

Sprenger, R. A. *Hygiene for Management*, 6th Edition. Doncaster, UK: Highfield Publications, 1993.

INDEX

A

Abortion and congenital illness, 41
Aerobes, 25
Aerobic, defined, 191
Africans
  susceptibility to food poisoning, 44
AIDs patients. *See* Higher-risk
  individuals
Alaska, botulism outbreaks, 69
Alcohol gels, 115
Alcoholism, 46
Alfalfa sprouts, *E. coli* poisoning, 61
Allergies, 20
Anaerobic bacteria, 25, 104
  defined, 191
Antacids, effect of, 124–25
Antibacterial cleaners, 116–17, 118,
  140
  defined, 191
Antibacterial soaps and wipes, 115, 139,
  140
Antibiotic resistance, 31–33
Antiseptic gel, 139–140
Apple juice, 61
Arthritis, diarrhea and, 40–41
Away from home, avoidance of food
  poisoning
  camping, 138–39
  food courts, 136
  picnics, 139–40
  potlucks and nonprofit events,
    141–42
  restaurants, 133–36, 137
  school lunches, 140–41
  street vendors, 136, 137
  traveling abroad, 137–38

B

Baby foods, refrigeration, 77
Bacillus
  heat-resistance, 21
  moisture and, 23
Bacillus cereus
  described, 165–66
  poisoning, described, 151, 153

Bacteria
  See also specific bacteria
  aerobes, 25
  anaerobic bacteria, 25, 104
  common types of, 17
  defined, 191
  generally, 16–17
  growth and multiplication of,
    20–25
    moisture, 23–24
    time bombs, 24–25
    warmth, 21–23
  guide to food poisoning terms,
    165–81
  heat-resistance, 21
  pathogenic bacteria, 16–17
Baked goods
  bakeries, 64–65
  home storage, 80
Barbecue cooking, 89
Bean sprouts, 61
Berries
  raspberries, 9, 28, 61
  strawberries, 61
Bleach, 116–17, 118, 140
Blood, infection in, 154–55
Body organs, infection in, 154–55
Body's defenses against food
  poisoning, 145–46
Bottled foods
  home storage, 79
  shopping for, 69, 70
Botulism
  See also Clostridium botulinum
  antitoxin, 151
  complications of, 40
  home preservation of foods, 103–5
  infants, 69
  science of, 151
Bovine spongiform encephalopathy
  (BSE)
  See also Creutzfeldt-Jakob
    disease (CJD)
  definition, 2
  described, 29–31

197

Bovine spongiform encephalopathy (BSE) (*Continued*)
prions and, 16
rise in poisoning, 10
Bread bins, self-service, 65
Breads. *See* Baked goods
Brucella abortus, 166–67
Brucella melitensis, 166
Brucellosis, 166–67
BSE. *See* Bovine spongiform encephalopathy (BSE)
Buffets, 94–95, 101

C

Camping, 138–39
Campylobacter infection
arthritis and, 40
described, 153–54
Guillain-Barré syndrome, 41–42
statistics on infected chickens, 47, 57
Campylobacter jejuni, 153–54
described, 167–69
Canada
botulism outbreaks, 69, 103, 151
bovine spongiform encephalopathy (BSE), 29–31
cattle, antibiotic resistant *Salmonella,* 31
parasitic worms, 19
Salmonella infection, outbreaks, 156
Salmonella typhimurium, 31
waterborne gastroenteritis, 29
Canned foods
dented cans, 69, 127
home canning. *See* Home preservation of foods
home storage, 79
shopping for, 68–69
Cantaloupes, *E. coli* poisoning, 61
Caribbean people
susceptibility to food poisoning, 44
Catering, 98–99
Cattle
antibiotic resistant *Salmonella,* 31
"hamburger disease." *See* *Escherichia coli* poisoning
"mad cow disease." *See* Bovine spongiform encephalopathy (BSE)

Causes of food poisoning, 11–25
allergies, 20
bacteria, growth and multiplication of, 20–25
chemicals, 12–13
environmental pollutants, 14–15
food intolerance, 20
germs, 15–19
naturally occurring poisons, 14–15
parasitic worms, 19–20
solid objects, 13–14
Check-out, shopping for food, 71
Cheese
pathogenic bacteria, 16
Salmonella infection, 155–56
Chemical contamination, 12–13
Chemotherapy, 45
Chicken
Salmonella infection, 26–27, 47
spit-roast chicken, delis, 63
statistics on infected chickens, 47, 57
Children. *See* Higher-risk individuals
Chocolate, *Salmonella* infection, 155–56
Cholera. *See* *Vibrio cholerae O1*
Ciguatoxins, 189
CJD. *See* Creutzfeldt-Jakob disease (CJD)
Clean, defined, 191
Cleaning and sanitation of kitchens. *See* Design and sanitation of kitchens
Cleansers, 116–17, 118
antibacterial cleaners, defined, 191
Clostridium
heat-resistance, 21
moisture and, 23
waterborne gastroenteritis, 29
Clostridium botulinum
See also Botulism
canned foods, 69
conditions for growth of, 104, 151
defined, 25
described, 169–70
detection of, 106
nervous system and, 40
Clostridium perfringens, 152, 170
Colon, described, 148
Color of food, 58–59

Complaints about conditions
shopping for food, 54–56
Complete Guide to Home Canning,
Preserving, and Freezing
(USDA), 103
Complications of food poisoning,
39–42
abortion and congenital illness, 41
arthritis, 40–41
Guillain-Barré syndrome, 41–42
hemolytic uremic syndrome
(HUS), 41
memory loss, 42
Contaminant, defined, 191
Cooking utensils, metals, 13
Corn syrup, infant botulism, 69
Counters, kitchen, 112, 116–17
Cows. *See* Cattle
Crabs, naturally occurring
poisons, 14
Creutzfeldt-Jakob disease (CJD) *See*
also Bovine spongiform
encephalopathy (BSE)
defined, 10
described, 29–31
Crock-pots, 86
Cross-contamination
avoidance of, 82, 83–84
defined, 191
Cryptosporidiosis, 18, 185
Cryptosporidium, 18–19, 44
Cryptosporidium parvum, 185
Cutting boards, 113–14
Cyclospora, 18–19, 28, 61
Cyclospora cayetanensis, 171, 184
Cyclospora poisoning, 9

D

Dairy foods
See also Cheese; Eggs; Milk
refrigeration, 76–77
Date stamps, 57, 58, 66, 127
Dehydration, 39
defined, 191
Delis, high-risk foods, 62–63
Design and sanitation of kitchens,
111–18
cleaning and sanitizing, 115–18
countertops, 116–17
equipment, 116

floors, 118
guidelines for, 118
home remedies, 129
sponges and dishcloths, 117
walls, 118
counters, 112, 116–17
cutting boards, 113–14
equipment, choice of, 114–15
cleaning equipment, 116
floors
cleaning, 118
design of, 113
food storage space, 112–13
handwashing and, 114–15
personal hygiene tips, 115
planning, 111–14
sinks, 112
soaps, 114–15
walls
cleaning, 118
design of, 113
Detergents, defined, 191
Developing countries, drinking
water, 18
Diarrhea
See also specific types of illness
berries, 28
drinking water and, 18–19, 137–38
higher-risk individuals, 38–39
Diarrhetic shellfish poisoning (DSP),
188
Diet, nutrition and, 46–47
Dietary factors increasing risk of
illness, 123–25
Digestive passage, 146–48
Dioxins, 14–15
Dishcloths, 117
Disposal of food, 96–97
preservation of foods, suspect cans,
107
Doggie bags, 135–36
Domoic acid, 189
Double dipping, 102
Dried foods, 24
home storage, 79
shopping for, 69–70
Drinking water
camping, 139
protozoa, 18–19
traveling abroad, 137–38

Drinks, shopping for, 69–70
DSP (diarrhetic shellfish poisoning),
    188
Dysentery
    foodborne dysentery, defined,
        192

E

E. coli poisoning. See Escherichia
    coli poisoning
Eggs
    baked goods, use in, 64
    preparing and cooking, 84
    Salmonella infection, 26–27, 84
    shopping for, 67
Egyptian mummies, bacteria, 22
Elderly. See Higher-risk individuals;
    Seniors, cooking for
England
        See also Great Britain; United
            Kingdom
    bovine spongiform encephalopathy
        (BSE), 29–31
    phenolic chemicals in water
        supply, 15
Enteric infections, defined, 191
Environmental pollutants,
    14–15
Environmental protection agency
    (EPA), 116
Epidemic cholera. See Vibrio
    cholerae O1
Equipment, kitchen
    choice of, 114–15
    cleaning equipment, 116
Escherichia coli poisoning
    fruit juices, 67
    "hamburger disease"
        causes of, 27
        described, 171–72
        increase in outbreaks, 2
        kidney failure, 7, 41, 148
        prevention of, 28
        recent outbreaks, 9
        verotoxins, 148
    O157, 59
        produce, linked to, 61
        statistics, 57
Europe
    cattle, antibiotic resistant
        Salmonella, 31

E. coli poisoning
    produce, linked to, 61
    Salmonella typhimurium, 31
    trichinosis, 20
    waterborne gastroenteritis, 29

F

Farm stands, food shopping, 54
Finger foods, 101–2
Fish. See Seafood
Floors, kitchen
    cleaning, 118
    design of, 113
Foodborne dysentery, defined, 192
Food courts, 136
Food intolerance, 20
Food poisoning, generally
    causes of. See Causes of food
        poisoning
    complications of. See
        Complications of food
        poisoning
    dealing with, 49–50
    defined, 192
    guide to food poisoning germs,
        165–89
    kitchen, prevention of food
        poisoning. See Kitchen,
        prevention of food poisoning
    rise of. See Rise of food poisoning
    symptoms of. See Symptoms of
        food poisoning
Food safety quiz, 159–64
Food storage space, kitchen,
    112–13
"Foreign bodies" in manufactured
    food, 13–14
Freezers. See Frozen foods
Frozen foods
    freezers, 77–78
    length of time to store, 78
    preservation of food, 109
    refreezing, 68, 100
    shopping for, 68
    thawing of, 68, 75, 78–79, 99
        microwave, 91
Fruit
        See also specific type of fruit
    contamination, 9, 28

Fruit juices, shopping for, 67
Fungi, defined, 14, 192

G

Gastroenteritis
  defined, 192
  Salmonella infection, 9–10
  waterborne protozoa, 28–29
Germs, 15–19, 148–50
  antibiotic resistance, 31–33
  bacteria. *See* Bacteria
  defined, 192
  guide to food poisoning germs. *See*
    Guide to food poisoning
    germs
  number needed to cause illness,
    149–50
  protection against, 155–56
  protozoa. *See* Protozoa
  signs of, 81
  variation in ability to cause illness,
    148–49
  viruses. *See* Viruses
Giardia, 18
Giardia lamblia, 186–87
Giardiasis, 18
Glossary, 191–94
Great Britain
    See also England; Scotland;
      United Kingdom
  inspections of food stores, 55
Grilling, 89
Ground beef
  "hamburger disease." *See*
    Escherichia coli poisoning
  purchase of, 58
Guide to food poisoning germs
  bacteria, 165–81
  parasites, 184–88
  seafood toxins, 188–89
  viruses, 181–83
Guillain-Barré syndrome, 41–42

H

"Hamburger disease." *See*
    Escherichia coli poisoning
Handwashing
  camping, 139

design and sanitation of kitchens,
    114–15
  picnics, 140
  preparing and cooking food, 82
Haricot beans, 14
Health, overall, 42–43. *See also*
    Higher-risk individuals
Hemolytic uremic syndrome
    (HUS), 41
Hepatitis A virus
  complications of, 40
  described, 181–82
  mollusks, 87
  strawberries, 61
Heredity, susceptibility to food
    poisoning, 44
Higher-risk individuals
  age and risk, 44
  alcoholism and, 46
  chemotherapy, 45
  cooking for
    dietary factors increasing risk of
      illness, 123–25
    foods to avoid, 121–22
    how to cook for, 122–23
  defined, 3
  diarrhea, 38–39
  infections, susceptibility to food
      poisoning, 44–45
  preexisting medical conditions, 45
  radiation therapy, 45
  raw foods and, 122
  severe symptoms, medical help, 49
  smokers, 46
  symptoms of food poisoning,
    38–39
  Toxoplasma, newborns, 41
  vomiting, 38–39
Histamine, defined, 192
Holidays and parties, cooking for,
    98–102
  buffets, 101
  catering, 98–99
  finger foods, 101–2
  home parties, 100–102
  turkeys, cooking, 99–100
Home, prevention of food poisoning.
    See Kitchen, prevention of food
    poisoning

Home preservation of foods, 69, 103–10
  botulism, prevention of, 103–5
  disposal of suspect cans, 107
  freezing, 109
  jams, jellies, and preserves, 108–9
  oils, flavored, 110
  pesto sauce, 110
  safety tips, 105–6, 108
  smoked foods, 109
  spoilage, signs of, 106–7
  techniques for
    heating without pressure, 107
    high-pressure canning, 105–7
    without heat, 109–10
Honey, infant botulism, 69
Horse meat, 20
Hot foods, cooling, 95–96
HUS. *See* Hemolytic uremic syndrome (HUS)

I

Iceberg lettuce, 61
Immune systems, depressed. *See* Higher-risk individuals
Immunity, defined, 192
Incubation period
  See also specific bacteria and viruses
  defined, 192
Infant botulism, 69
Infants. *See* Higher-risk individuals
Infections, susceptibility to food poisoning, 44–45
Instant-read thermometers, 85, 94
Interrupted cooking, 86
Intestines
  infection in, 153–54
  poison (toxin) produced in, 152–53
Investigations by public health officials, 50
Irradiation of foods, 123

J

Jack In The Box restaurants, 9
Jams, jellies and preserves
  home preservation, 108–9
Japan, *E. coli* poisoning, 61

K

Kidney failure
  "hamburger disease," 41, 148
  hemolytic uremic syndrome (HUS), 41
Kitchen, prevention of food poisoning
  design and sanitation. *See* Design and sanitation of kitchens
  disposal of food, 96–97
  higher-risk individuals, cooking for
    dietary factors increasing risk of illness, 123–25
    foods to avoid, 121–22
    how to cook for, 122–23
  holidays and parties, cooking for, 98–102
    buffets, 101
    catering, 98–99
    finger foods, 101–2
    home parties, 100–102
    turkeys, cooking, 99–100
  hot foods, cooling, 95–96
  leftovers, 95–96, 152
  potlucks and nonprofit events, for, 141–42
  preparing and cooking food, 82–92
    barbecue, 89
    cross-contamination, avoidance of, 82, 83–84
    eggs, 84
    grill, 89
    handwashing, 82
    marinating food, 83
    microwave cooking, 90–92
    mollusks, 87
    partial or interrupted cooking, 86, 152
    raw foods of animal origin, 82–83
    recipes, modifying for safety, 88
    safety tips, 86–87
    slow cooking, 86
    tasting, 88
    temperature for cooking, 84–86
  preservation of foods, 103–10
    botulism, prevention of, 103–5
    disposal of suspect cans, 107
    freezing, 109

jams, jellies, and preserves,
   108–9
oils, flavored, 110
pesto sauce, 110
safety tips, 105–6, 108
smoked foods, 109
spoilage, signs of, 106–7
techniques for, 105–10
refrigeration. *See* Refrigeration
reheating cooked food, 96
school lunches, 140–41
serving food, 93–94
specific germs, safety measures
   against
   Bacillus cereus, 166
   Brucella abortus, 167
   Campylobacter jejuni, 168–69
   Clostridium botulinum, 170
   Clostridium perfringens, 170
   Cryptosporidium parvum, 185
   Cyclospora cayetanensis, 171, 184
   E. coli poisoning, 172
   Giardia lamblia, 187
   hepatitis A virus, 182
   Listeria monocytogenes, 173
   Norwalk-like virus, 183
   Salmonella, 175
   Salmonella paratyphi, 176
   Salmonella typhi, 176
   Shigella, 177
   Staphylococcus aureus, 178
   Trichinella spiralis, 188
   Vibrio cholerae O1, 178
   Vibrio parahaemolyticus, 180
   Vibrio vulnificus, 180
   Yersinia enterocolitica, 181
spoiled food, signs of, 80–81
storing food, 75–81
   baked goods, 80
   bottled food, 79
   canned food, 79
   dried foods, 79
   fruits and vegetables, 79–80

L

Large intestine, described, 148
Leftovers, dealing with, 95–96, 152
   seniors and single persons, 128
Lifestyle, susceptibility to food
   poisoning and, 45–46

Listeria
   pregnancy and, 43
   salads, prepackaged, 62
   temperatures and, 23
Listeria monocytogenes, 173
Listeriosis, 173
Lobsters, naturally occurring
   poisons, 14

M

"Mad cow disease." *See* Bovine
   spongiform encephalopathy
   (BSE)
Malnutrition, 46–47
Marinating food, 83
Market stalls, food shopping, 54
Meats
   See also Chicken; Ground beef;
      Turkey
   baked goods, fillings, 64
   "hamburger disease." *See*
      Escherichia coli poisoning
   horse meat, 20
   shopping for
      fresh meat, 57–60
      organic meat, 59–60
   stamps, meat and poultry, 59
Memory loss, 42
Menu planning, seniors and single
   persons, 127
Meringue, 64
Metals, potentially dangerous, 13
Microbe, defined, 192. *See also*
   Germs
Microwave cooking, 90–92
   materials and packaging, 91–92
   seniors and single persons, 127
   thawing, 91
Milk, shopping for, 67
Milwaukee, waterborne
   gastroenteritis outbreak, 29
Minnesota, *Salmonella*
   gastroenteritis, 9–10
Moisture
   bacteria, growth and multiplication
      of, 14, 23–24
Molds, 81
Moldy food, 81
Mollusks, cooking, 87
Mouth, described, 146

Mycotoxins, 81
  defined, 192

N

Naturally occurring poisons, 14–15
Neurotoxic shellfish poisoning, 189
Neutralizing defenses, 156
North America. *See* Canada; United
  States
Norwalk-like virus, 183
Nutrition and diet, 46–47

O

Offal, defined, 193
Oils, flavored, 110
Oral rehydration, 39
Orange juice contamination, 13
Oysters, 87

P

Packaging
  leaky packages, 58
Paper towels, 116–17, 118
Paralytic shellfish poisoning (PSP),
  188
Parasites
  See also specific parasite
  defined, 193
  guide to food poisoning germs,
    184–88
  worms, parasitic, 19–20
Partial cooking, 86, 152
Parties, cooking for. *See* Holidays
  and parties, cooking for
Pasteurization
  Cryptosporidium and, 19
  defined, 193
  germ counts, reduction of, 123
Pastries. *See* Baked goods
Pathogen, defined, 193
Pathogenic bacteria, 16–17
PCBs, 14–15
Pesto sauce, 110
Phage type
  defined, 193
Phenolic chemicals, 15
Picnics, 139–40
Plankton, defined, 193

Potlucks and nonprofit events,
  141–42
Poultry. *See* Chicken; Turkey
Power outages, freezers and, 77–78
Preexisting medical conditions, 45
Pregnant women, *Listeria* and, 43
Preparing and cooking food. *See*
  Kitchen, prevention of food
  poisoning
Preservation of foods, home. *See*
  Home preservation of foods
Prions, 16
Produce
  See also Fruit
  E. coli poisoning linked to, 61
  home storage, 79–80
Protozoa
  defined, 193
  generally, 18–19
PSP (paralytic shellfish poisoning),
  188
Public health officials, 50

Q

Quiz, food safety, 159–64

R

Radiation therapy, 45
Raspberries, 9, 28, 61
Raw foods
  animal origin, of, cooking and
    preparation, 82–83
  beans, 14
  eggs, 26–27, 84
  higher-risk individuals and, 122
  restaurants, 135
  risks, 124
  viruses and, 18
Recipes, modifying for safety, 88
Reconstituted dried foods, 24
Refreezing of frozen foods, 68, 100
Refrigeration
  defined, 193
  frozen foods. *See* Frozen foods
  home, 75–79
    baby foods, 77
    correct temperatures, 23, 75–76
    dairy foods, 76–77
  length of time to store foods, 78

market stalls, 54
stores and supermarkets, 65–67
Reheating cooked food, 96
Reporting food poisoning illness, 49–50
Restaurants, 133–36
  choice of foods, 135
  doggie bags, 135–36
  take-out foods, 136
  traveling abroad, 137
  visual clues, 134–35
Rise of food poisoning, 7–10
  statistics, 8–9

S

S. enteritidis, 26
Sabotage of food, deliberate, 70
Salad bars, 63–64
Salads, prepackaged, 62
Salmonella
  described, 174–75
  moisture and, 23–24
Salmonella infection
  antacids and, 124–25
  arthritis and, 40
  baked goods, 64
  chickens, 26–27
  described, 153, 154
  eggs, 26–27, 84
  foods associated with, 24
  increase in outbreaks, 2, 155–56
  Minnesota, gastroenteritis outbreak, 9–10
  number of germs needed to cause, 150
  statistics on infected chickens, 57
Salmonella paratyphi
  described, 175–76
Salmonella typhi, 155
  complications caused by, 40
  contracting of, 17
  described, 175–76
  effect of, 149
Salmonella typhimurium
  antibiotic resistance, 31
Sanitation and design of kitchens. See Design and sanitation of kitchens
Sanitize, defined, 193
School lunches, 140–41

Science of food poisoning, 145–56
  blood, infection in, 154–55
  body organs, infection in, 154–55
  body's defenses against food poisoning, 145–46
  digestive passage, 146–48
  food, poison (toxin) produced in, 150–51
  germs, 148–50. See also Germs
  intestines
    infection in, 153–54
    poison (toxin) produced in, 152–53
Scombrotoxin poisoning, 15, 188
Scotland, rise of food poisoning, 8–9
Scrapie, sheep, 29–30
Seafood
  See also Shellfish
  antibiotics, commercial fish farming, 33
  environmental pollutants, 14–15
  fishy smell, 60
  freshness of, 15
  guide to food poisoning germs, 188–89
  shopping for, 60–61
  toxins, 60
Seals, bottled foods, 69
Self-assessment, 159–64
Self-service
  bread bins, 65
  salad bars, 63–64
Seniors, cooking for
  cleaning and disinfection, home remedies, 129
  immune system, changes in and traditional foods, 128–29
  leftovers, dealing with, 128
  menu planning, 127
  microwaving, 127
  shopping, 126–27
Serving of food, 93–95
  buffets, 94–95
  two-hour rule, 93–94
Sheep, scrapie, 29–30
Shelf life, defined, 194
Shellfish
  See also Seafood
  contaminated, 47
  naturally occurring poisons, 14

Shigella
  arthritis and, 40
  described, 176–77
Shigellosis. *See Shigella*
Shopping for food
  bakeries, 64–65
  bottled foods, 69, 70
  canned foods, 68–69
  check-out, 71
  color of food, 58–59
  date stamps, 57, 58, 66, 127
  delis, 62–63
  dried food and drinks, 69–70
  leaky packages, 58
  meat, selection of, 57–60
    organic meat, 59–60
  meat and poultry stamps, 59
  odor of food, 58–59
  refrigerated foods, 65–67
    frozen foods, 68
  salad bars, 63–64
  seafood, selection of, 60–61
  seniors and single persons,
      126–27
  transporting of food, 71
  where to shop, 53–56
    farm stands, 54
    food staff, observing, 54
    inspections of food stores,
        55–56
    market stalls, 54
    proactive behavior, 54–56
    visual clues, 53–54
Sickle cell disease, 44
Single persons, cooking for
  cleaning and disinfection, home
      remedies, 129
  leftovers, dealing with, 128
  menu planning, 127
  microwaving, 127
  shopping, 126–27
Sinks, kitchen, 112
Small intestine, described, 147
Smoked foods, preservation of, 109
Smoking, tobacco, 46
Sneeze-guards, 63
Soaps, kitchen, 114–15
Solid objects in food and drink,
    13–14
South America
  fruit, contamination, 28

Species, defined, 194
Spleen, 45
Spit-roast chicken, delis, 63
Sponges, kitchen, 117
Spore, defined, 194
Squirrels
  bovine spongiform encephalopathy
      (BSE), 29
Staphylococcus
  moisture and, 23
  temperature and, 86
Staphylococcus aureus, 150–51
  described, 177–78
Sterilization, defined, 194
Stomach, described, 146–47
"Stomach flu," 38
Strain, defined, 194
Strawberries, hepatitis A virus, 61
Street vendors, 136, 137
Stress, 45
Symptoms of food poisoning, 37–39
  coping with mild symptoms,
      48–49
  defined, 194
  dehydration, 39
  elderly, 38–39
  infants and children, 38–39
  severe symptoms, medical help, 49
  "stomach flu," 38

T

Taenia tapeworms, 19
Take-out foods, 136
Tampering with food, deliberate, 70
Tapeworms, 19
Tasting, when cooking, 88
Temperatures
  bacteria, growth and multiplication
      of, 21–23
  cooking, 84–86
    internal cooking temperatures,
        85, 100
  hot foods, cooling, 95–96
  microwave cooking, 90–91
  refrigeration, 23, 75–76
Tetrodotoxin, 189
Thermometers
  cooking, 85
  refrigerators, 76
  serving food, 94

Thermoses, 141
Toxins, defined, 194
Toxoplasma, newborns, 41
Transporting of food, 71, 142
Traveling abroad, 137–38
    drinking water, 137–38
    restaurants, 137
    street vendors, 137
Trichinella spiralis, 40
    described, 187–88
Trichinosis, 19–20
    See also Trichinella spiralis
    complications of, 40
Turkeys, cooking, 99–100
Two-hour rule, serving of food,
    93–94
Typhoid fever, 17, 149, 155
    complications of, 40

U

Undercooked foods
    "hamburger disease." *See*
        Escherichia coli poisoning
    restaurants, 135
United Kingdom
    See also England; Great Britain;
        Scotland
    bovine spongiform encephalopathy
        (BSE), 10
    parasitic worms, 19
    rise of food poisoning, 8, 10
    Salmonella infection, chocolate,
        156
    Salmonella typhimurium, 31
United States
    antibacterial cleansers, 116
    berries, diarrhea and, 28
    botulism outbreaks, 69, 103, 151
    cattle, antibiotic resistant
        Salmonella, 31
    inspections of food stores, 55
    parasitic worms, 19
    rise of food poisoning, 8–10

Salmonella infection, outbreaks,
    156
Salmonella typhimurium, 31
    waterborne gastroenteritis, 29
United States Department of
        Agriculture (USDA), 57, 59
    *Complete Guide to Home Canning,
        Preserving, and Freezing,* 103

V

Vegetables. *See* Produce
Verotoxins, 148
    defined, 194
Vibrio cholerae O1, 178–79
Vibrio parahaemolyticus, 179–80
Vibrio vulnificus, 180
Viruses
    See also specific virus
    defined, 194
    generally, 17–18
    guide to food poisoning germs,
        181–83
Vomiting
    See also specific types of illness
    higher-risk individuals, 38–39

W

Walls, kitchen
    cleaning, 118
    design of, 113
Warmth
    growth and multiplication of
        bacteria, 21–23
Water
    See also Drinking water
    consuming large amounts of, 124
    waterborne protozoa, 18–19
        gastroenteritis and, 28–29
Wooden cutting boards, 113–14

Y

Yersinia, 40
Yersinia enterocolitica, 180–81
Yogurt, pathogenic bacteria, 16

ABOUT THE AUTHORS

Elizabeth Scott is a microbiologist specializing in consumer hygiene issues and is one of only a few people who have a working knowledge of the subject in North America, Britain, and Europe. Scott has both a master's degree and a Ph.D. in microbiology and has spent twenty years researching, teaching, and advising in the field of food and environmental hygiene in both commercial and consumer sectors. She has published many scientific papers on aspects of hygiene in the home and the prevention of foodborne illness, and she is a regular contributor at national and international conferences. For many years, Scott was involved in informing the British public about food hygiene via public-speaking engagements, television, radio, and press articles. She moved to the United States in 1993 and now has professional interests on both sides of the Atlantic. During 1995, she appeared on *Good Morning America* with advice on how to avoid cross-contamination in the kitchen, and her work was featured in a *Washington Post* article on germs in the home. She continues to make television appearances and give advice on preventing food poisoning at home. Scott is currently working as a consultant in food and environmental hygiene and lives with her husband and three sons in Newton, Massachusetts.

Paul Sockett, Ph.D., has over twenty-five years' experience in the fields of microbiology and epidemiology. For fourteen years, he worked as a principal scientist at the Communicable Disease Surveillance Centre in England, where he had responsibility for the production of a weekly United Kingdom report on communicable disease. More recently, he was responsible for the surveillance of foodborne disease in England and Wales. Sockett has published papers on infectious disease surveillance and on the epidemiology and economic impact of foodborne disease, and he is a frequent speaker at national and international meetings. While in the

United Kingdom, he contributed regularly to teaching programs and served on various working groups concerned with the prevention of foodborne illness. He recently moved to Canada where he lives with his wife and three children. At present, he works for the Laboratory Centre for Disease Control, Health Canada, where he is involved in the development of surveillance programs for infectious diseases, including enteric food and waterborne diseases.